Understanding Pregnancy

A Doctor-Mother's Perspective on Pregnancy, Birth, and Early Motherhood

— and Everything In Between —

Author

Dr. Babita Das

MBBS, MS (Obstetrics & Gynaecology)

Your doctor. Your guide. Your friend through every week.

Dr. Chandrabhan Rajoria

First Edition, 2025 | Published in India

Published by - Dr. Babita Das

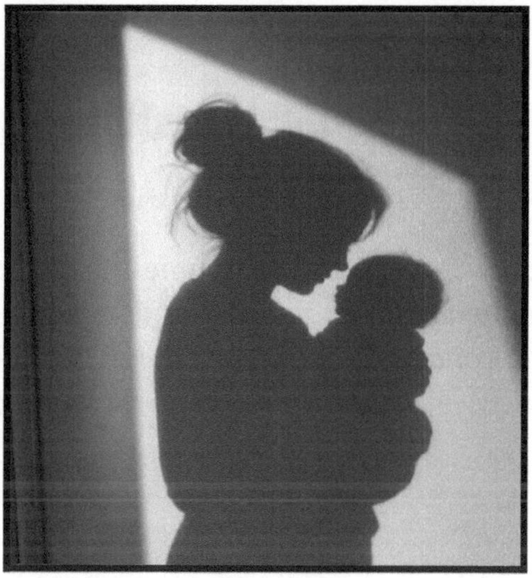

Medical Disclaimer

This book is a guide and companion; it is not a replacement for your own doctor's advice. Every pregnancy is unique. If anything concerns you, please speak to your healthcare provider. Trust your instincts. You know your body.

Acknowledgements

I am deeply grateful to my school teachers, undergraduate faculty at BMC Sagar, postgraduate faculty at GRMC Gwalior, my respected PG guide, and every patient who contributed to my learning and professional growth. I extend my heartfelt thanks to my husband, Dr Chandrabhan Rajoria, whose unwavering support, encouragement, and dedication have stood beside me in every endeavor.

Becoming a mother enriched my understanding of pregnancy beyond textbooks and clinical practice, providing invaluable insights into the physical, emotional, and social aspects of this remarkable journey.

This book reflects my experiences from conception to returning to professional life, combined with evidence based medical knowledge. It is written not only for expectant mothers but also for families, caregivers, healthcare professionals, students, and everyone involved in maternal care. Through greater awareness and shared knowledge, we can work together to improve maternal health, promote safer pregnancies, and ensure better outcomes for mothers and their families.

For every woman who has ever held a pregnancy test with trembling hands.

For the woman who has waited years for this moment. For the one who is terrified. For the one who is alone. For the one surrounded by too many opinions from too many relatives. For the one navigating two jobs and morning sickness at the same time. For the one who has lost before and is trying again with cautious, hopeful heart.

You are not alone. I have walked this road with thousands of women. Now I am walking it with you.

— Dr. Babita Das

A Letter to You

Dear Reader,

If you are pregnant, planning a pregnancy, or supporting someone through this beautiful journey, welcome. I am glad you are here.

As an obstetrician, I have cared for thousands of mothers over the years. Despite different backgrounds, their questions were often the same: "Is this normal?" "Should I worry?" "What is happening to my baby?" This book is my attempt to answer those questions in a simple, clear, and trustworthy way.

This is not a medical textbook. It is a practical guide that combines scientific knowledge, years of clinical experience, and my own journey through pregnancy. During my pregnancy, I realized that even as a doctor, I needed reassurance, support, and honest conversations. That experience gave me an even deeper respect for every mother.

In our society, many women hesitate to talk openly about pregnancy, body changes, emotions, and their concerns. My hope is that this book will replace fear and myths with knowledge and confidence.

Pregnancy is a remarkable journey. My aim is to help you understand it with clarity, confidence, and peace of mind.

Let us begin this journey together.

With best wishes,

Dr. Babita Das

Table of Content

1

Before the Journey Begins

Planning, Trying, and the Two-Week Wait

Thinking About Getting Pregnant

So you are thinking about it. Maybe you have been thinking about it for a while, having quiet conversations with your partner after dinner, pausing at the baby clothes section of a shop you had no intention of stopping at, noticing children at family gatherings in a way you never quite did before. Or maybe the decision has arrived less gradually: a birthday has passed, a close friend has had her second baby, or your mother-in-law has graduated from gentle hints to what can only be described as a sustained campaign.

However you have arrived at this moment, this chapter is for you. Because the months before pregnancy the pre-conception period are among the most medically significant in the entire journey. And most women receive no guidance about them at all.

When a woman attends her first antenatal appointment, usually around 8 to 10 weeks of pregnancy she is already nearly three months into one of the most critical developmental periods of her baby's life. The embryonic period, during which every major organ system is formed from scratch, begins at fertilisation and ends at 8 weeks. By the time most women know they are pregnant, the neural tube has closed (or not), the heart has begun to beat, and the foundations of the brain, spine, kidneys, liver, and limbs are being laid down , all in the complete absence of any medical input, advice, or monitoring.

Pre-conception care is the attempt to make that unmonitored period as safe as possible. It is the gift you can give your future baby before either of you knows the journey has started.

✍ My NOTE

I have been practising obstetrics for 5 years. In that time, I have noticed something consistently: the women who arrive at their first antenatal visit having already started folic acid, having already had their anaemia treated, having already reviewed their medications these women tend to have smoother pregnancies. Not because they have been lucky, but because they have been prepared. Preparation is the most powerful thing you can do.

The One Thing You Must Do Right Now

Before we discuss anything else, I need you to do one thing. If you are reading this while planning a pregnancy or while trying to conceive, or while wondering whether you might already be pregnant please go and buy folic acid today.

Folic acid is a B vitamin. Your developing baby needs it during the very first days of existence, before you could possibly know you are pregnant,to correctly close the neural tube, the embryonic structure that becomes the brain and spinal cord. This closure happens between days 21 and 28 after conception. It happens silently, invisibly, while you are going about your life. And without adequate folic acid in your system at that precise moment, the tube can fail to close completely, resulting in spina bifida (incomplete closure at the spine) or anencephaly (absence of most of the brain). These are serious, largely irreversible conditions.

They are also largely preventable.

A daily dose of 400 micrograms (0.4 mg) of folic acid started at least one month before conception and continued through the first twelve weeks of pregnancy, reducing the risk of neural tube defects by 50 to 70 percent. This is one of the clearest, most consistent findings in all of preventive medicine. Folic acid tablets cost almost nothing at any medical shop in India. There is no reason not to start today.

Women at higher risk , those who have previously had a pregnancy affected by a neural tube defect, those taking anticonvulsant medications (particularly valproate or carbamazepine), those with diabetes, obesity, or malabsorption conditions ,should take 5 mg daily, available on prescription.

Your Pre-Conception Checklist

A pre-conception visit with your gynaecologist , ideally two to three months before you plan to start trying , is the most efficient way to address all of the following. But even without a formal visit, here is what matters:

Have Your Blood Tested

Several blood tests are worth doing before pregnancy, rather than waiting until after:

- Haemoglobin / Full blood count: Iron-deficiency anaemia affects more than 50% of Indian women of reproductive age. In pregnancy, it increases the risk of preterm birth, low birth weight, and postpartum haemorrhage. It is far easier to correct before pregnancy than during it. A haemoglobin below 12 g/dL in a non-pregnant woman deserves investigation and treatment.
- Thyroid function (TSH): Hypothyroidism is the most common hormonal condition in women of reproductive age, and it is frequently undiagnosed. Untreated hypothyroidism can impair fertility, increase the risk of miscarriage, and if it persists into pregnancy, is associated with neurodevelopmental delay in the child. A TSH above 2.5 mIU/L in a woman planning pregnancy is worth treating with levothyroxine, under your doctor's guidance.
- Blood group and Rh factor: If you are Rh negative and your partner is Rh positive, your baby may be Rh positive, which can cause antibody problems in current or future

pregnancies. Knowing this in advance allows for proper planning and prophylaxis.

- Fasting blood glucose or HbA1c: Undiagnosed pre-diabetes or type 2 diabetes at the time of conception is a significant risk factor for birth defects, particularly cardiac and neural tube defects, because organogenesis happens before most women start monitoring their blood sugar in pregnancy. Screen now, treat now.
- Rubella IgG: If you are not immune to rubella (German measles), you should receive the MMR vaccine at least one month before attempting conception. Rubella infection in the first trimester causes severe congenital defects (deafness, heart disease, cataracts).
- Vitamin D: As discussed at length later in this book, Vitamin D deficiency is extraordinarily prevalent in India, affecting 70-90% of women in many studies, and is associated with impaired fertility, miscarriage, pre-eclampsia, and poor fetal bone development. Check your 25-OH Vitamin D level. Supplement if below 30 ng/mL.
- Haemoglobin electrophoresis: Essential for women from communities with a high prevalence of thalassaemia or sickle cell disease, which includes many parts of India, particularly Maharashtra, Gujarat, West Bengal, Odisha, and tribal populations across the subcontinent. If you carry a haemoglobin abnormality, your partner should also be tested. If both partners are carriers of the same condition (for example, both beta-thalassaemia carriers), each pregnancy has a 25% chance of producing an affected child. Genetic counselling before conception gives you choices.

Review Your Medications

Some commonly used medications are unsafe in pregnancy and must either be stopped or switched to safer alternatives before conception. This is a conversation to have with your doctor never stop prescribed medication without medical advice, but the categories to be aware of include:

- ACE inhibitors and ARBs (used for hypertension and kidney disease, e.g. enalapril, lisinopril, losartan, valsartan): Can cause fetal renal damage and oligohydramnios in the second and third trimesters. Switch to labetalol, nifedipine, or methyldopa before conception.
- Valproate (used for epilepsy and bipolar disorder): Associated with a 6-10% risk of major congenital malformations and a significant increase in neurodevelopmental delay in children. Every woman of reproductive age taking valproate should have a documented discussion with her neurologist or psychiatrist about alternatives.
- Isotretinoin (Accutane, Roaccutane, used for severe acne): Highly teratogenic. Requires two forms of contraception during treatment and for one month after stopping. Do not attempt conception until at least one month after the last dose.
- Methotrexate (used for rheumatoid arthritis, psoriasis, and other conditions): Teratogenic and can cause miscarriage. Stop at least three months before attempting conception; ensure folate stores are replenished.
- Warfarin (blood thinner): Teratogenic in the first trimester. Requires switching to low-molecular-weight heparin at the time of conception.

Lifestyle Changes That Actually Matter

There is a great deal of advice floating around about pre-conception lifestyle, some of it useful and some of it not. Here is the evidence-based version:

- Stop smoking ,completely, not just reduce. Smoking impairs fertility in both men and women, increases the risk of ectopic pregnancy, miscarriage, placental complications, preterm birth, low birth weight, and sudden infant death syndrome. There is no safe level of smoking in pregnancy. If you need help stopping, ask your doctor about nicotine replacement therapy or prescription support.

- Stop alcohol — completely. Alcohol is a teratogen, a substance proven to cause birth defects. Fetal alcohol spectrum disorders represent a continuum of brain damage caused by prenatal alcohol exposure, and there is no established safe level. The safest approach is no alcohol from the time you start trying.
- Reduce caffeine to a moderate level. In pregnancy, the recommended maximum is 200 mg per day, approximately one strong coffee or two to three cups of tea. High caffeine intake before and during early pregnancy has been associated with increased miscarriage risk. Beginning to moderate your intake before conception is sensible.
- Achieve a healthy weight if possible. Both underweight (BMI below 18.5) and obesity (BMI above 30) are associated with impaired fertility and increased obstetric risk. Women with a BMI above 30 have significantly elevated risks of gestational diabetes, hypertensive disorders, and caesarean section, as well as increased difficulty achieving conception. Even a 5-10% reduction in weight can meaningfully improve fertility and pregnancy outcomes in overweight women.
- Exercise regularly. Women who exercise regularly before and during pregnancy have shorter labours, lower rates of gestational diabetes, better mental health, and easier postpartum recovery. Walking, swimming, yoga, any moderate regular activity is beneficial. Extreme exercise or crash dieting immediately before conception is not recommended as it depletes nutritional reserves.

" **Suman's Story**

"My husband and I had been trying for eight months," Deepa told me when she came for a pre-conception check. "I thought something was wrong with me." Her haemoglobin was 9.2 g/dL — severely anaemic. Her TSH was 6.8 — hypothyroid. Her Vitamin D was undetectable. She had been taking an ACE inhibitor for mild hypertension since her twenties. None of this was her fault; no one had ever told her these things mattered for conception. We treated her anaemia, started thyroid medication, supplemented her Vitamin D, and switched her blood pressure tablet. She conceived four months later. Her pregnancy was uncomplicated. She still sends me mithai every Diwali.

Understanding Your Menstrual Cycle

To make a baby, you need to have intercourse at the right time which means understanding when you ovulate. In a textbook 28-day cycle, ovulation occurs around day 14. But textbook cycles are exactly that: textbook. Real women have cycles of 21 to 35 days, cycles that vary month to month, and cycles affected by stress, illness, travel, and the full chaos of ordinary life. For many women, day 14 is not ovulation day at all.

The fertile window is approximately six days long: the five days before ovulation plus the day of ovulation itself. Sperm can survive in the female reproductive tract for up to five days in favourable conditions, while the egg is viable for only 12 to 24 hours after ovulation. This means that intercourse in the two to three days before ovulation is often more effective than intercourse on the day itself.

How to Find Your Fertile Window

There are several methods, each with different advantages:

Ovulation Predictor Kits (OPKs) detect the LH (luteinising hormone) surge that triggers ovulation approximately 24 to 36 hours before it happens. You will see a positive result, a smiley face on digital kits, a line as dark as or darker than the control on strip kits. The day of the positive OPK and the following day are your peak fertile days. OPKs are available at pharmacies throughout India at modest cost and are the most reliable home method for timing intercourse.

Cervical mucus monitoring involves paying attention to the natural vaginal discharge that changes in character throughout the cycle. In the days before and around ovulation, fertile-quality mucus is produced: clear, slippery, stretchy, resembling raw egg white. This mucus facilitates sperm transport through the cervix. Outside the fertile window, mucus is thick, opaque, sticky, or absent. When you see the egg-white consistency, your fertile window is open.

Basal body temperature (BBT) charting involves taking your temperature first thing every morning, before getting out of bed or speaking or drinking anything, using a basal thermometer. After ovulation, progesterone causes a sustained temperature rise of 0.2 to 0.4 degrees Celsius that lasts until your next period. Because this rise occurs after ovulation has happened, BBT is most useful in retrospect, to identify when you ovulated this cycle and thereby predict the next cycle. Used alongside cervical mucus monitoring, it provides a comprehensive picture.

For women with very irregular cycles, polycystic ovary syndrome (PCOS), or a history of difficulty conceiving, a transvaginal ultrasound follicle-tracking series performed by your gynaecologist is the most accurate method of identifying the fertile window. It is not necessary for most women, but is invaluable when simpler methods are not giving clear results.

How Often to Try

The evidence is clear: intercourse every one to two days during the fertile window gives the highest chance of conception per cycle. Daily intercourse is not significantly more effective than every-other-day, and for some couples, the pressure of daily sex transforms an intimate act into a clinical obligation, which can create stress that counterproductively affects both libido and ovulation. My advice: identify your fertile window, make love during it because you want to, and do not turn your bedroom into a laboratory.

✍ My NOTE

The question I am asked most often by newly married couples trying to conceive is: "What position is best?" The honest answer is that there is no scientific evidence that any sexual position improves the chances of conception. Gravity does not play a meaningful role in fertilisation. Lying still afterwards for 15 minutes has been suggested in some studies to very modestly improve conception rates, but the effect is small. Enjoy the process. That matters more than any position.

For Your Partner

This is a chapter that most pregnancy books forget to write, and I think that is a significant omission. Male factor infertility contributes to approximately 40 to 50 percent of all infertility cases. Yet the expectation that men will be involved in pre-conception care, the assumption that what a man does with his body before conception has any relevance, is still poorly established in most societies, including India.

It does matter. Sperm quality is affected by lifestyle, health, and environment in ways that are directly modifiable. And because sperm take approximately 74 days to mature (the process of spermatogenesis), the effects of changes made today will be reflected in sperm quality in about three months. Which means that now is an excellent time for your partner to:

- Stop smoking: Smoking reduces sperm concentration, motility, and morphology — all three of the parameters assessed in a semen analysis. Male smokers have significantly lower fertility than non-smokers.
- Reduce or stop alcohol: Heavy alcohol consumption reduces testosterone and impairs sperm production. Moderate consumption has a less clear effect, but given that alcohol is being stopped anyway for the woman, it is a supportive and sensible gesture for the partner to do the same.
- Avoid heat exposure: Spermatogenesis requires a temperature approximately 2 to 4 degrees Celsius lower than core body temperature — which is why the testes are located outside the body. Prolonged hot baths, saunas, laptop heat on the lap, very tight underwear, and sedentary work with poor ventilation can all raise scrotal temperature and impair sperm production. Switch to loose cotton underwear. Take short warm showers rather than long hot baths.
- Maintain a healthy weight: Obesity in men is associated with reduced testosterone, impaired sperm parameters, and increased DNA fragmentation in sperm.
- Review medications: Anabolic steroids (used for bodybuilding) profoundly suppress spermatogenesis and can cause azoospermia (complete absence of sperm) — which may take months to years to recover after stopping. Certain antihypertensives, antidepressants, and other medications also affect fertility.
- Eat a good diet: Antioxidants — Vitamin C, Vitamin E, zinc, selenium, coenzyme Q10 — support sperm quality by reducing oxidative stress. These are obtained from fresh fruits, vegetables, nuts, seeds, and lean protein. A diet of processed food, excessive red meat, and refined carbohydrates is associated with poorer sperm parameters.

If you have been trying to conceive for twelve months (or six months if you or your partner is over 35), request a semen analysis. It is a simple, non-invasive test. It should be done at the same time as initial female fertility investigations — not as an afterthought after months of testing the woman.

The Two-Week Wait

The "two-week wait" is the informal name for the 10 to 14 days between ovulation and the earliest reliable pregnancy test — the period during which you cannot yet know whether conception has occurred. It has its own particular quality of suspended time: every morning you wake up and wonder. Every twinge of your abdomen gets noted and interrogated. Every slight shift in your mood or appetite becomes potential evidence.

I want to save you from a great deal of unnecessary anxiety about this period by telling you something important: almost all of the "symptoms" that women experience during the two-week wait — breast tenderness, bloating, slight nausea, fatigue, emotional sensitivity, cramps — are driven by progesterone, which rises after ovulation regardless of whether fertilisation has occurred. They are identical whether you are pregnant or not. You cannot symptom-spot your way to a reliable answer. The only reliable answer is a pregnancy test.

Home pregnancy tests detect hCG — human chorionic gonadotrophin — the hormone produced by the embryo after implantation. Most tests can detect hCG from the day of a missed period, and some sensitive tests can detect it a day or two before. Test with your first morning urine, which is the most concentrated. Read the result in the time window specified by the test manufacturer (usually 3 to 5 minutes).

A faint line is a positive. hCG levels are simply low in early pregnancy; a faint line does not mean a weak pregnancy. If you are unsure, test again in two days — the line will be darker as hCG doubles. A truly negative test — no line at all — means either the test is too early, or this was not the month.

And if it was not the month: this is normal. Even in a healthy couple with no fertility concerns, at peak fertility, the probability of conception in any given cycle is approximately 20 to 25 percent. Most healthy couples conceive within six months of trying. Patience — however difficult — is warranted.

" Ritu's Two-Week Wait

"I tested on day 8," Ritu told me, laughing at herself. "And then on day 9. And then day 10. I bought seventeen tests. My husband said we were supporting the pharmaceutical industry." She came in at 7 weeks pregnant, having eventually, mercifully, seen a positive result at day 14. "Why does no one tell you that it is this agonising?" she asked. I told her: because if we told you in advance, no one would ever go through it. The hope is stronger than the anxiety. That is why people try again.

✔ WHAT TO DO THIS WEEK

✔ Start folic acid 400 mcg daily — right now, before conception

✔ Book a pre-conception check with your gynaecologist

✔ Check haemoglobin, thyroid function (TSH), Vitamin D, blood group

✔ Review all medications with your doctor — some are unsafe in pregnancy

✔ Stop smoking and alcohol

✔ Check rubella immunity — vaccinate if not immune (wait 1 month before trying)

✔ If you have a family history of thalassaemia or sickle cell: both partners should be screened

✔ Use OPKs to identify your fertile window

✔ Encourage your partner's pre-conception health check

✔ Test on the day of your missed period — not before

2

The First Trimester

Weeks 1 to 13: The Secret Months

The first trimester is the trimester nobody talks about and yet it contains some of the most profound events of the entire pregnancy. It is the trimester of secrets: the secret that you are pregnant, the secret your body is keeping about the extraordinary work it is doing, and sometimes the secret of your own emotional complexity about this enormous change that is beginning.

It is also the trimester of the couch. Of lying down when you get home from work. Of apologising to your husband for not cooking dinner and then feeling too guilty to go to sleep. Of pretending to be fine at your desk when you are actually counting the minutes until you can go somewhere private and be sick.

This trimester is hard. And it is miraculous. And both of those things are true at the same time.

WEEKS 1 & 2

The Invisible Beginning

In the curious convention of obstetric dating, you are not yet pregnant in weeks 1 and 2. Pregnancy is counted from the first day of your last menstrual period — the date everyone knows and can report accurately — rather than from the date of conception, which almost no one knows precisely. This means that the first two "weeks of pregnancy" are actually the week of your period (week 1) and the week your body is preparing to ovulate (week 2).

The reason for this system is entirely practical. The last menstrual period (LMP) is a reliable landmark. The date of conception is usually a guess. When clinicians need to calculate a due date, estimate gestational age, or make management decisions, a consistent, reproducible starting point matters more than a physiologically precise one.

So technically: you are not pregnant yet. You are preparing. Somewhere in your ovaries, a cohort of follicles is responding to rising FSH (follicle-stimulating hormone) from your pituitary gland, growing toward maturity. One follicle — the dominant follicle — will outgrow the others. By the end of week 2, it will rupture, releasing an egg that has been developing since before you were born.

THE SCIENCE BEHIND IT

The Egg That Has Been Waiting

The egg released at your ovulation this cycle began developing when you were a fetus in your own mother's womb. Every egg a woman will ever release was present in an arrested, immature state at the time of her birth.

At birth, a female infant has approximately 1 to 2 million oocytes. By puberty, this number has fallen to around 300,000 through a process of natural attrition called atresia. Of these, approximately 400 will ever be ovulated across a reproductive lifetime. The rest continue to atrophy, this process of declining egg number and quality is the biological basis of the fertility decline associated with advancing age.

This is also why maternal age affects egg quality: older eggs have been sitting in their arrested state for longer, accumulating damage. The higher rate of chromosomal abnormalities in pregnancies of older women, including Down syndrome , is primarily a consequence of this accumulated chromosomal instability in the egg, not in the sperm.

WEEK 3

Fertilisation and the Journey Home

Week 3 is when the story truly begins. Somewhere in the ampullary portion of your fallopian tube — the wide outer section near the ovary — an egg and a sperm have found each other. This meeting, after a journey of extraordinary improbability (of the 200 to 500 million sperm deposited in the vagina, only a few hundred ever reach the fallopian tube, and only one successfully fertilises the egg), produces a zygote: a single cell containing 46 chromosomes — 23 from you and 23 from your partner — that will become your child.

In the next three to four days, the zygote divides as it travels along the fallopian tube toward the uterus. It becomes a 2-cell embryo, then 4-cell, then 8-cell, and by the time it arrives in the uterine cavity, a morula — a solid ball of 16 cells. Fluid then begins to accumulate within the morula, creating a central cavity, and it becomes a blastocyst: a hollow sphere of approximately 100 cells, with an inner cell mass (which will become the baby) and an outer layer called the trophoblast (which will become the placenta).

By day 6 to 10 after fertilisation, the blastocyst lands on the uterine lining and begins to implant. The trophoblast cells invade the endometrium, burrowing in. And as they do, they begin producing hCG — the hormone that will sustain this pregnancy, prevent menstruation, and eventually show up as a positive line on a pregnancy test.

♥ YOUR BABY RIGHT NOW

Week 3: A single cell, then two, then four...

Your baby is currently smaller than the full stop at the end of this sentence. She is a tiny ball of dividing cells, rolling slowly along your fallopian tube. She has no features, no heartbeat, no visible form. And yet she already has everything that makes her genetically unique: her chromosomes are set, her blood type is determined, and if she carries a Y chromosome, she is already biologically male. She is arriving home.

♡ WHAT YOU MIGHT BE FEELING

- Almost certainly nothing — it is too early for any symptoms
- Possibly a very slight implantation cramping as the blastocyst embeds in the uterine lining — many women mistake this for the beginning of a period
- Light spotting in some women — "implantation bleeding" — typically lighter and shorter than a period, and often brownish rather than bright red
- The quiet absence of anything: no period coming, but no confirmation yet either

WEEK 4

The Test

Your period is due this week. In its place, you may find yourself staring at a small plastic stick that is about to tell you something life-changing.

A positive pregnancy test means hCG has reached detectable levels in your urine — typically above 20 to 25 mIU/mL. Most home pregnancy tests achieve this sensitivity on the day of a missed period. Some "early response" tests claim accuracy from 4 to 6 days before the missed period, though false negatives are more common at this stage simply because hCG levels are still very low.

If the test is positive: the line may be faint. That is okay. A faint line is a positive line. hCG levels double approximately every 48 hours in early pregnancy, so a faint line today will be a much darker line in two days. Sit with the news. Let it be real. Feel whatever you feel — excitement, terror, disbelief, joy, overwhelm, all of the above simultaneously — without judgment. There is no correct emotional response to a positive pregnancy test.

Then: start your folic acid if you have not already. Make an appointment with your gynaecologist for your booking visit at around 8 to 10 weeks. And — if you have been drinking alcohol — stop immediately. Today is day one.

If the test is negative and your period does not arrive: wait 48 to 72 hours and test again with fresh first-morning urine. Sometimes hCG has not yet reached detectable levels at the time of the first test. If tests remain negative after a week of missed period, see your doctor — there are other reasons for missed periods, and if you are pregnant, a blood test will be able to confirm it even before the urine test is positive.

♥ YOUR BABY RIGHT NOW

Week 4: About 0.1–0.2 mm — the size of a poppy seed

The blastocyst is fully implanted in your uterine wall. The inner cell mass is differentiated into the three primary germ layers — ectoderm, mesoderm, and endoderm — from which every tissue and organ of the human body will form. The amniotic sac is beginning to form around the embryo. The yolk sac — which will serve as the embryo's first source of nutrients and blood cells — is visible on ultrasound as a small ring. The trophoblast is dividing aggressively, forming the early placenta. Your body is completely unrecognisable to itself at the cellular level, even if nothing is visible from the outside.

♡ WHAT YOU MIGHT BE FEELING

- A missed period — the first sign for most women
- Breast tenderness — often one of the earliest symptoms, caused by progesterone
- Fatigue — a profound, bone-deep tiredness that is unlike ordinary tiredness
- Mild nausea may begin for some women, though many feel nothing yet
- Increased urination — hCG increases renal blood flow, even at this early stage
- Emotional sensitivity — inexplicable tearfulness is genuinely common this early
- An odd sense of "something has changed" that you cannot quite articulate

✔ WHAT TO DO THIS WEEK

✔ Take a home pregnancy test with first morning urine

✔ If positive: start folic acid 400 mcg immediately

✔ Stop alcohol completely — from today

✔ Book your 8-10 week antenatal appointment

✔ Tell your partner — if and when you are ready

✔ Do not yet tell everyone else — many women wait until after the NT scan at 12-13 weeks

✔ Do not Google every symptom — you will regret it

" The Two Lines

"I tested at 11 p.m. because I could not sleep," Pooja told me at her booking visit. "My husband was already asleep. I stood in the bathroom for twenty minutes just staring at it. I did not wake him up. I went back to bed and lay there in the dark thinking: am I actually going to be a mother? And then at 2 a.m. I woke him up and showed him and we both sat there in the dark together not saying anything, because there was nothing to say, really. It was already everything."

WEEKS 5 & 6

When the Body Speaks

Weeks 5 and 6 are when the pregnancy stops being a private secret between you and a plastic test and starts being a physical reality that your body insists upon announcing — to you, if not to the world. Nausea. Fatigue. Breast tenderness that makes walking up stairs uncomfortable. The sudden and violent dislike of things you previously loved.

One of my patients described the transition from week 4 to week 6 as follows: "Monday I was a normal person. By Thursday I could not be in the same room as fried onions." This is not unusual. The first trimester has a way of rearranging your relationship to the physical world.

♥ YOUR BABY RIGHT NOW

Weeks 5–6: 3–6 mm — the size of a lentil or small pea

Something extraordinary has happened in the past week: your baby has a heartbeat. Not a fully formed four-chambered heart — that comes later. What is beating right now is a primitive cardiac tube that has formed and begun to pulse at approximately 100 to 130 beats per minute. On a transvaginal ultrasound at 6 weeks, this flicker is visible — a tiny, rhythmic movement that is the first visible evidence of a life distinct from your own. The neural tube — the precursor to the brain and spinal cord — is closing. Tiny arm and leg buds have appeared, like small paddles on either side of the embryonic disc. The embryo is curved, seahorse-shaped, and already more complex than anything our ancestors could have imagined.

Everything About the Nausea

Nausea and vomiting of pregnancy — dubbed "morning sickness" by someone who had evidently never experienced it after noon, or in the afternoon, or at 9 p.m. while watching television — affects approximately 70 to 80 percent of pregnant women. For roughly half of those women, it involves actual vomiting. For 0.5 to 2 percent, it becomes severe enough to require medical treatment.

Understanding why it happens helps — even if the understanding does not make it easier.

The primary driver of pregnancy nausea is hCG. This hormone rises steeply in the first trimester, peaking at around 8 to 10 weeks — which is exactly when nausea is at its worst for most women. hCG is structurally similar to TSH (thyroid-stimulating hormone) and stimulates thyroid function, leading to a transient mild hyperthyroidism in many pregnant women. The thyroid connection may partially explain the nausea. hCG may also act directly on the area postrema — the brain's vomiting centre. In addition, progesterone slows gastric emptying and relaxes the lower oesophageal sphincter, making reflux more likely.

What this means practically: nausea is worst when the stomach is empty (because there is nothing to buffer the increased acid production), worst when hCG is rising (which is also when you are most anxious about the pregnancy, compounding the nausea), and worst in the morning (because you have been fasting for 8 hours overnight). And it usually — not always, but usually — begins to improve as hCG levels plateau at around 10 to 12 weeks.

What Helps — An Honest Assessment

Here is what actually works, in approximate order of evidence:

- Never let your stomach go completely empty. Keep dry crackers, plain biscuits (Marie biscuits, toast without butter), or a few plain rice puffs by your bedside and eat them before you even sit up in the morning. Eating something small every two hours — even when eating feels impossible — reduces nausea more than anything else.
- Ginger: The evidence is genuine. In randomised controlled trials, ginger in doses of around 1 gram per day consistently reduced nausea scores in pregnant women. Adrak chai (without too much milk if dairy is a trigger), ginger water, ginger biscuits, sucking a small piece of raw ginger — all are options. Ginger powder capsules 250 mg four times daily are the dose used in most trials.
- Cold foods and cold drinks: Hot food has stronger aromas, which often trigger nausea. Cold foods — cold dahi, cold fruit, cold plain rice — are often better tolerated. Room-temperature or cold water is better than hot beverages for many women.
- Nimbu paani: A classic Indian remedy that genuinely works — the lemon provides Vitamin C and has a genuinely anti-nausea effect; the salt and sugar replace electrolytes lost through vomiting. Squeeze half a lemon into a glass of cool water with a pinch of rock salt (sendha namak) and a teaspoon of sugar. Sip slowly.
- Pyridoxine (Vitamin B6): 10 to 25 mg three times daily. Safe, modestly effective, available at any pharmacy. Often used as the first-line pharmacological intervention before moving to prescription anti-emetics.
- Lemon: The smell of fresh lemon has a documented anti-nausea effect. Keep a halved lemon in a small container. Inhale it when nausea strikes. This is not folklore; it has been tested.
- Small, frequent meals instead of three large ones: Your stomach is already working slower than usual. Large meals sit in it for longer, producing more acid, causing more reflux and nausea. Six to eight small snacks throughout the day is far better than three standard meals.

- Acupressure wristbands (P6 point): The evidence is mixed, but they carry no risk and some women find them helpful. Available at pharmacies.
- Rest: Fatigue dramatically worsens nausea. If you can rest in the afternoon, do. Sleep is medicine in the first trimester.
- Fresh air: Many women find that spending time outdoors — even simply sitting near an open window — helps. The smell of the outside world is often less triggering than indoor cooking smells and confined spaces.

When to Call Your Doctor About Nausea

Nausea that is manageable with the above measures, even if miserable, does not require medical attention — though you absolutely can and should discuss it at your antenatal appointment. However, some situations do require a call:

⚠ Call Your Doctor About Nausea If:

- You cannot keep any fluids down for more than 12-24 hours
- You are urinating very little or very dark urine (sign of dehydration)
- You feel dizzy, faint, or significantly weak
- You are losing weight rapidly
- You have abdominal pain alongside the vomiting (this may indicate something other than pregnancy nausea)
- The nausea is so severe it is making normal life impossible

Hyperemesis Gravidarum (HG) is a medical diagnosis — severe pregnancy nausea requiring hospital treatment. IV fluids, electrolyte replacement, and anti-emetic medication make an enormous difference. You do not have to endure it. Ask for help.

✍ My NOTE

One more thing about nausea: please do not apologise for it. I have patients who come in looking hollowed out — they have not eaten a proper meal in three weeks, they are surviving on plain biscuits and lemon water — and they say, "I'm sorry, I know I'm being dramatic." You are not being dramatic. You are experiencing a real physiological phenomenon that medicine has sometimes been slow to take seriously. Your symptoms are real. Your suffering is real. And relief is available.

♡ WHAT YOU MIGHT BE FEELING

- Nausea — from mild queasiness to debilitating vomiting, and everything in between
- Profound fatigue — the kind where climbing stairs feels like a significant achievement
- Extreme breast tenderness — even a bra strap can be uncomfortable
- Food aversions — sudden, violent dislike of foods you previously enjoyed
- Heightened sense of smell — you may smell things no one else can detect, and they may all be terrible
- Increased urination
- Mild abdominal bloating
- Emotional volatility — tears over small things, irritability, sudden waves of anxiety
- The strange experience of having a secret this large and being unable to share it

WEEKS 7 & 8

A Human Being Is Taking Shape

Weeks 7 and 8 represent one of the most astonishing periods in human development. Your embryo is still tiny — smaller than a kidney bean — but in these two weeks, the cellular blueprint is being executed with breathtaking precision. Every major organ system of the human body is forming simultaneously, from a template encoded in chromosomes so small they cannot be seen with the naked eye.

This is why the first trimester — despite its invisibility to the outside world — deserves so much respect. What is happening inside you right now makes every engineering project in human history look simple.

♥ YOUR BABY RIGHT NOW

Weeks 7–8: 13–20 mm — the size of a kidney bean or small grape

Your baby has a face. Dark spots where eyes are forming, nostril pits beginning to take shape, the earliest hint of a chin and cheekbones. Tiny paddle-like hands are developing digits — ridges that will become fingers. The intestines have grown so rapidly that the abdominal cavity cannot yet contain them; they loop out temporarily into the umbilical cord — this is completely normal and will resolve when the abdomen has grown large enough. The heart is beating at 150 to 170 beats per minute — faster than an adult heart, because a small heart must beat more rapidly to move blood efficiently. The brain is the fastest-growing structure: every minute, approximately 250,000 new neurons are being produced.

Your Booking Appointment

Your first formal antenatal appointment — the booking visit — should happen between 8 and 10 weeks. It is the longest and most comprehensive appointment of your entire pregnancy, and it establishes the foundation for everything that follows. Come prepared: bring any previous medical records you have, a list of all medications you take (prescription and over-the-counter), and ideally your partner.

At this visit, your doctor will:

- Take a detailed medical history — your health background, any chronic conditions, previous pregnancies and their outcomes, family history of genetic conditions, mental health history, and social circumstances
- Take an obstetric history — any previous pregnancies, miscarriages, terminations, caesarean sections, preterm births, or complications
- Measure your blood pressure and weight (to establish your baseline — blood pressure readings in pregnancy are only meaningful if you know what your blood pressure normally is)
- Perform or arrange an ultrasound scan — to confirm the pregnancy is in the uterus (not ectopic), to see the heartbeat, to measure the gestational age, and to check for twins
- Arrange a panel of booking blood tests
- Discuss the antenatal care schedule, antenatal classes, and the options for prenatal screening
- Answer your questions — and you should have questions. Write them down before you go.

Booking Blood Tests — What They Are and Why

The list of blood tests at the booking visit looks intimidating. Here is a plain-language explanation of each one:

Full blood count: Checks your haemoglobin level (anaemia screen), white blood cells (infection indicator), and platelets (clotting). In India, anaemia is found in over 50% of pregnant women. Your haemoglobin needs to be at least 11 g/dL — ideally above 12 g/dL — to safely sustain pregnancy, labour, and delivery.

Blood group and Rh type: Your ABO blood group and whether you are Rh positive or Rh negative. If you are Rh negative and your partner is Rh positive, your baby may be Rh positive. If any of the baby's blood enters your circulation — through the placenta, at delivery, or through a bleed — your immune system may develop antibodies against Rh-positive blood. In a subsequent pregnancy, these antibodies can cross the placenta and destroy a Rh-positive baby's red blood cells (haemolytic disease of the fetus and newborn). This is largely preventable with anti-D immunoglobulin injections given during and after pregnancy.

Thyroid function (TSH): Hypothyroidism, even mild, is associated with miscarriage, preterm birth, and neurodevelopmental delay in the child. A TSH above 2.5 mIU/L in the first trimester warrants treatment with levothyroxine.

Blood glucose or HbA1c: To screen for pre-existing diabetes — which, as discussed, carries significant first-trimester risks because it affects organogenesis. Some doctors prefer to do a full oral glucose tolerance test (OGTT) at this stage for high-risk women.

HIV: Offered routinely to all pregnant women with appropriate counselling. Mother-to-child transmission of HIV is reduced to less than 2% with antiretroviral therapy — but only if HIV-positive status is known. Knowing is life-saving.

Hepatitis B surface antigen (HBsAg): If positive, your baby will need hepatitis B vaccine and immunoglobulin at birth to prevent transmission. Chronic hepatitis B in the mother is also associated with worsening liver function during pregnancy.

VDRL or RPR (syphilis screen): Congenital syphilis — infection of the baby with Treponema pallidum — can cause stillbirth, severe disability, and death. It is entirely treatable with penicillin. Screening early allows treatment early.

Rubella IgG: If you are not immune and have not been vaccinated, you will be offered vaccination after delivery. During pregnancy, if you are exposed to rubella (German measles), your doctor needs to know you are not immune so that appropriate assessment and counselling can be provided.

Haemoglobin electrophoresis: In Indian populations with significant thalassaemia carrier frequency, this is important. If you are found to be a carrier, your partner should also be tested.

Urine culture: Asymptomatic bacteriuria — bacteria in the urine without any symptoms — affects approximately 5% of pregnant women and, if untreated, can progress to kidney infection (pyelonephritis), which is associated with preterm labour. A simple urine culture identifies and allows treatment of this silent condition.

♡ WHAT YOU MIGHT BE FEELING

- Nausea may be at or near its peak this week
- Fatigue that does not respond to sleep — a different, deeper tiredness than usual
- Food aversions and smell sensitivities often at their worst
- Possible heartburn beginning – progesterone relaxes the lower oesophageal sphincter
- Waistline thickening slightly, though no visible bump yet
- Emotional intensity – moments of profound joy followed by inexplicable anxiety
- The first scan – seeing the heartbeat for the first time – often produces an emotional response that surprises even the most composed people

✔ WHAT TO DO THIS WEEK

✔ Attend your booking visit (8-10 weeks) – this is the most important appointment of the first trimester

✔ Have all booking blood tests done as requested

✔ Take your iron and folic acid supplement every day

✔ If your TSH is elevated, start levothyroxine as directed

✔ Rest whenever you can – fatigue is your body's instruction to slow down

✔ Begin to think about who you will tell and when

✔ Write down your questions before each appointment – you will forget them otherwise

WEEKS 9 & 10

Becoming a Fetus

At nine completed weeks — 63 days from the first day of your last menstrual period — your baby undergoes a change in name that reflects a genuine developmental transition. The embryonic period is over. The embryo becomes a fetus.

The distinction is not merely semantic. During the embryonic period, the body's major structures were being established from scratch, from three layers of cells, in an environment of extraordinary vulnerability to insult. From week 9 onwards, the fetal period begins: a period of growth, maturation, and refinement of systems already established. The risk of structural birth defects from external insults — teratogens — drops significantly. The pregnancy is becoming more stable.

For many women, this week also brings something else: the first, cautious beginning of belief. You have seen the heartbeat on the scan. You have heard it confirmed in blood tests and measurements. You may still be holding your breath. But something is beginning to shift from anxious hope to settled reality.

♥ YOUR BABY RIGHT NOW

Weeks 9–10: 30–40 mm — the size of a small strawberry or grape

Your baby looks unmistakably human. She has a forehead, an upper and lower jaw, tiny earlobes, and nostrils. Her fingers and toes are fully separated — the webbing between them has dissolved. She has begun to make spontaneous movements: bending, flexing, even something like a startle response, all quite invisible to you for now as she is far too small for you to feel. Her diaphragm is forming. Her intestines, which had been herniated into the umbilical cord, are returning to the abdominal cavity. Her heartbeat, now at around 170 to 180 beats per minute, is visible — and audible on a Doppler — at every visit from now.

The First Trimester Scan — What You Will See

Your first ultrasound — the dating scan, usually performed between 7 and 10 weeks — may be a transvaginal scan (a thin probe placed in the vagina, which gives clearer images at this stage) or a transabdominal scan (the probe on the abdomen), or both.

The sonographer will measure the crown-rump length (CRL) — the distance from the top of the head to the bottom of the rump — to establish the gestational age precisely. This measurement is most accurate in the first trimester; after 14 weeks, individual size variation makes it less reliable as a dating tool. If the CRL measurement significantly differs from dates calculated from your LMP, the scan dates will usually be used instead — this is not a cause for concern, simply a reflection of normal variation in ovulation timing.

You will be able to see the heartbeat flickering. You will be able to see the yolk sac — a round structure providing nutrients before the placenta is fully functional. If you are having twins, this is usually when it is first identified.

The scan may also identify a subchorionic haematoma — a collection of blood between the placenta and the uterine wall, visible as a dark area near the pregnancy. These are common, found in about 2% of first trimester ultrasounds, and most resolve spontaneously without any treatment. Your doctor will explain its size and whether it is clinically significant.

✍ My NOTE

The first scan is an emotional experience for almost every couple, regardless of how composed or medically informed they are. I have seen professors of medicine cry when they hear the heartbeat. I have seen women who have been through multiple pregnancies go completely still and quiet the first time they see the movement on screen. There is something in that moment — seeing something that is yours, that is real, that is alive — that bypasses all rationality. Give yourself permission to feel it.

WEEKS 11, 12 & 13

The End of the Beginning

You have almost made it through the first trimester. And as you approach its end, you may notice several things changing, both physically and emotionally.

For many women, week 12 or 13 brings a marked improvement in nausea. This is not your imagination. As hCG levels plateau and begin to decline slightly, the nausea that it drives often eases considerably. Energy may begin to return. The extreme emotional volatility of the first weeks may settle. You may start to feel, for the first time in weeks, recognisably like yourself.

This is also the time of the NT scan — one of the most significant diagnostic appointments of the entire pregnancy.

♥ YOUR BABY RIGHT NOW

Weeks 11–13: 55–80 mm — the size of a fig or lime

Your baby now has fingernails and toenails. She is swallowing amniotic fluid and her kidneys are producing urine — which is added back to the amniotic fluid, creating a cycle she will maintain for the rest of the pregnancy. Her eyes, previously on the sides of her head like a fish, have moved to the front of her face. Her ears have reached their final position. She has the hiccup reflex. She can open and close her hands. She has taste buds. The external genitalia are differentiating — male babies are beginning testosterone production, causing the genital tubercle to develop into a penis. Female babies are developing ovaries containing the eggs that will, decades from now, potentially produce the next generation. On the NT scan, she may be seen rolling, stretching, and bouncing — the movements of a baby who has no idea yet how closely she is being watched.

The NT Scan, Your Most Important First Trimester Appointment

The nuchal translucency (NT) scan is performed between 11 weeks 0 days and 13 weeks 6 days — not before, not after. The timing matters because the NT measurement is only valid within this window. Book it as soon as you know you want it, because the booking slots fill up and the window closes.

The NT is a fluid-filled space at the back of the fetal neck. All fetuses have some fluid here; the question is how much. A larger NT is associated with a higher probability of chromosomal abnormalities — particularly Down syndrome (Trisomy 21), Edwards syndrome (Trisomy 18), and Patau syndrome (Trisomy 13) — as well as major cardiac defects.

NT measurement alone is not a screening test. It is combined with two blood markers — free beta-hCG (elevated in Down syndrome) and PAPP-A (reduced in Down syndrome) — and your age and gestational age, to generate a combined risk calculation. This "combined first-trimester screen" detects approximately 85 to 90% of Down syndrome cases at a 5% false-positive rate.

The result will be expressed as a probability — for example, "1 in 850" means the risk of Down syndrome is 1 in 850, which is low risk. "1 in 50" means the risk is higher. The cut-off for "high risk" is typically 1 in 150 or 1 in 300, depending on the laboratory. A high-risk result does not mean your baby has Down syndrome. It means the probability is elevated enough to warrant further investigation.

NIPT — The More Accurate Option

Non-invasive prenatal testing (NIPT) uses a blood sample from the mother to analyse fragments of placental DNA (cell-free fetal DNA, or cfDNA) circulating in the maternal bloodstream. It can be performed from 10 weeks of pregnancy. It has dramatically higher accuracy than the combined screen:

- Down syndrome (Trisomy 21): Detection rate over 99%, false positive rate below 0.1%
- Edwards syndrome (Trisomy 18): Detection rate approximately 97%
- Patau syndrome (Trisomy 13): Detection rate approximately 92%
- Sex chromosome abnormalities (Turner syndrome, Klinefelter syndrome): Detection rates 90-95%

NIPT is more expensive than the combined screen and is not yet universally available in public sector facilities in India. But its accuracy is such that major obstetric bodies worldwide — including FOGSI — now recommend offering it as a first-line screening option to all women, not just those over 35.

An important point: NIPT is a screening test, not a diagnostic test. A positive NIPT result means the probability of the condition is very high — but confirmation requires an invasive diagnostic test (CVS or amniocentesis) before irreversible decisions can be made.

THE SCIENCE BEHIND IT

What Down Syndrome Actually Is

Down syndrome is caused by the presence of three copies of chromosome 21 (trisomy 21) rather than the usual two. In 95% of cases, this occurs due to a random error during the formation of the egg — a failure of chromosome 21 to separate correctly during meiosis (non-disjunction). Because this error becomes more common as eggs age, the prevalence of Down syndrome increases with maternal age.

At age 25: approximately 1 in 1,500 births

At age 30: approximately 1 in 900

At age 35: approximately 1 in 350

At age 40: approximately 1 in 100

At age 45: approximately 1 in 30

People with Down syndrome have intellectual disability of varying severity, characteristic facial features, and a higher prevalence of congenital heart defects, thyroid disorders, and other conditions. They also have considerable strengths, capacities, and potential for joyful, meaningful lives. The range of outcome is wide.

If the NT or NIPT raises concern for Down syndrome, a confirmatory diagnostic test (amniocentesis or CVS) is offered. Couples who receive a confirmed diagnosis are offered genetic counselling and full information about the condition before making any decision about the pregnancy.

♡ WHAT YOU MIGHT BE FEELING

- Nausea beginning to ease for many women — a genuine relief
- Energy starting to return — many women emerge from the first trimester feeling dramatically better
- The bump becoming subtly visible, particularly at the end of week 13
- Excitement about telling people — you are approaching the conventional announcement window
- Possibly: a profound sense of transition from fear to cautious, growing confidence
- Nervousness about the NT scan — this is universal and completely understandable
- The first stirrings of wanting to talk to your baby, which you may find surprising

✔ WHAT TO DO THIS WEEK

✔ Book your NT scan immediately — the window is 11+0 to 13+6 weeks and it fills up

✔ Have the NT blood test at the same time (or just before) the scan

✔ Discuss NIPT with your doctor if you would like a more accurate chromosomal screen

✔ Start thinking about who you will tell and when

✔ Consider announcing the pregnancy after the NT scan — most major pregnancy guidance suggests this is the conventional "safe" point

✔ If your nausea has improved, take the opportunity to eat more nutritiously

✔ Begin walking or gentle exercise if you have not been active — the second trimester energy surge is coming

✔ Book the 20-week anatomy scan (18-22 weeks)

" Sunita's NT Scan

"The number came back as 1 in 55," Sunita told me, holding her husband's hand. Her voice was steady, but her knuckles were white. "My mother has been on the phone all day. My sister-in-law says it definitely means something is wrong." I asked her to sit. I explained: 1 in 55 means a probability of approximately 1.8%. That sounds alarming. But it also means a 98.2% probability that the baby does not have Down syndrome. The NT result had triggered the screening system correctly — this was a result that warranted further investigation, not a diagnosis. Sunita had NIPT. The result was low-risk for all conditions. She exhaled a breath it seemed she had been holding for two weeks. Her son was born full term, healthy and vigorous, and she named him after her husband's grandfather who had always been, she said, "a bit of a worrier."

3

The Second Trimester

Weeks 14 to 27: The Golden Months

Welcome to what many women describe as the best part of pregnancy. The worst of the nausea has usually passed. The crushing first-trimester fatigue has lifted. Your bump is beginning to show — and with it, a visible confirmation of something you have been carrying internally, in both senses, for three months. The world begins to respond to your pregnancy. Strangers smile. Colleagues offer their seats. Your mother-in-law suddenly finds herself possessed of opinions about your diet, your footwear, and whether you should be taking the stairs.

And then, somewhere around week 18 to 22, something happens that changes everything: you feel your baby move for the first time. It is the moment when the pregnancy transforms from a concept into a relationship.

WEEKS 14 & 15

Coming Into the Light

The second trimester begins officially at week 14. For most women, the transition from first to second trimester is palpable: a lifting of the fog, a return of appetite, a reconnection with the world outside the bedroom and the bathroom. If the first trimester was the pregnancy you kept secret from everyone including yourself, the second is the pregnancy you begin to inhabit.

Your uterus has risen out of the pelvis and into the lower abdomen. You may be able to feel it — a firm, rounded area a few centimetres below your navel, distinctly different from the soft tissue surrounding it. By week 15, it reaches approximately halfway between your pubic bone and navel.

The risk of miscarriage, which was highest in the first trimester, has dropped significantly. In a pregnancy where a heartbeat has been confirmed on scan at 12 weeks, the ongoing risk of loss is approximately 1%. This is not zero, but it is low enough that most women feel they can begin to let themselves believe.

♥ YOUR BABY RIGHT NOW

Weeks 14–15: 85–100 mm — the size of a lemon

Your baby can now make facial expressions — frowning, squinting, perhaps even a primitive smile as facial muscles respond to nerve impulses. She is practising breathing movements, inhaling and exhaling amniotic fluid to develop her lung muscles, though no gas exchange is happening through the lungs yet. She is responding to light — if a bright light is shone near your abdomen, she will move away from it. Her lanugo — fine, downy body hair — is beginning to cover her skin, keeping her warm in the amniotic fluid. She is almost constantly moving, though you cannot yet feel it. Her bones are hardening as calcium is incorporated. Her liver is producing bile. Her pancreas is producing insulin.

♡ WHAT YOU MIGHT BE FEELING

- For most women: a significant improvement in energy
- Return of appetite — and sometimes a substantial one
- Round ligament pain — sharp, brief stabbing pains on one or both sides of the lower abdomen when you move suddenly. Completely normal and harmless.
- Your waistline is disappearing — clothes that fitted last month may not fit this week
- Skin changes beginning: some women notice the linea nigra (dark line down the abdomen), darkening of the areolae, or changes in skin texture
- Headaches — common in the second trimester due to increased blood volume and hormonal changes. Paracetamol is safe. Stay well hydrated.
- Possible dizziness, particularly when standing up quickly — the blood pressure drop of pregnancy reaching its nadir

✍ A NOTE FROM DR. BABITA

Round ligament pain is one of the symptoms that generates the most panic calls in the second trimester. "Sharp pain on my right side, Doctor, could it be appendicitis?" The distinction: round ligament pain is brief (a few seconds), stabbing, triggered by sudden movement, and disappears almost immediately when you stop moving. Appendicitis pain is persistent, worsens over hours, and is accompanied by fever, nausea, and loss of appetite. If in doubt, call your doctor — but the vast majority of sudden, fleeting second-trimester abdominal pains are round ligament spasm. Slow down your movements. That is the entire prescription.

✔ WHAT TO DO THIS WEEK

✔ Enjoy the return of energy — use it to establish healthy habits that will serve you in the third trimester

✔ Start regular moderate exercise if you have not: walking 30 minutes daily, swimming, prenatal yoga

✔ Eat iron-rich foods at every meal — nausea is no longer an excuse

✔ Begin thinking about your birth plan — what you want, where you want to give birth, who you want present

✔ Tell your employer if you have not already — maternity leave planning should begin now

✔ Book your 20-week anatomy scan

✔ Consider a dental check-up – pregnancy gingivitis is real and deserves treatment

✔ Start wearing comfortable, supportive footwear – your centre of gravity is shifting

WEEKS 16 & 17

First Movements

Somewhere between week 16 and week 22, for first-time mothers, and often slightly earlier for women who have been pregnant before, one of the most extraordinary moments of pregnancy will happen: you will feel your baby move for the first time.

There is no way to prepare you for this adequately. There is no description that quite captures the quality of the experience. But let me try.

It does not feel like a kick. Not yet. The first movements are subtle — a fluttering, like the wings of a moth. A bubbling sensation, like carbonated water somewhere deep. A soft thud, as if someone has tapped you very gently from the inside. Some women describe it as feeling like a small fish turning just below the surface. Others compare it to the briefest possible muscle twitch, but in the wrong location for a muscle twitch.

The first time it happens, you may not be sure. You might think: was that it? And then it happens again, slightly differently, and you know. There is nothing else in the body that feels like this.

Write down the date. This is called "quickening" — from an Old English word meaning "alive" — and it marks the moment when the abstract knowledge of pregnancy becomes a physical, relational reality. From this point forward, your baby is not just a scan image or a heartbeat on a monitor. She is a presence, here, communicating with you through movement in the only way she can.

♥ YOUR BABY RIGHT NOW

Weeks 16–17: 110–130 mm — the size of an avocado

Your baby is now capable of hearing. Her inner ear structures are complete and functional — she can detect sounds both from within your body (your heartbeat, the gurgling of your digestive system, the sound of blood flowing through the placenta — a constant, rushing hum that is the soundtrack of her existence) and from outside (voices, music, the sounds of daily life filtered through amniotic fluid). Research consistently shows that newborns recognise and prefer the sound of their mother's voice — the voice they have been hearing for months. She is also developing her sense of taste, receiving flavours from the amniotic fluid she swallows, which is itself flavoured by what you eat. Studies show that babies exposed to certain flavours in utero show preference for those flavours after birth.

WEEKS 18–22

The Anatomy Scan

The mid-trimester anomaly scan — commonly called the "20-week scan" though it is performed anywhere between 18 and 22 weeks — is the most comprehensive ultrasound assessment of your entire pregnancy. It is an hour, sometimes longer, of systematic examination of your baby's anatomy: every major structure, measured and assessed against established norms.

For most women, the anomaly scan is an experience of wonder: seeing your baby in detail, watching her move, perhaps finding out her sex if you choose to know. For approximately 1 in 50 women, the scan identifies something that requires further investigation — a finding that was not expected. I want to prepare you for both possibilities.

♥ YOUR BABY RIGHT NOW

Weeks 18–22: 140–190 mm — the size of a large mango or small aubergine

Your baby is developing rapidly and is now perfectly proportioned, though still thin — she will begin laying down significant subcutaneous fat in the third trimester. Her face is beautiful: lips, eyelids, the distinctive shape of her nose. She has the tiny whorls of fingerprints. She is swallowing amniotic fluid, digesting it, and passing it as meconium — a dark green, sticky substance that accumulates in her bowel and will be her first "bowel movement" after birth. She is sleeping in cycles of about 20 to 30 minutes, alternating with periods of activity. At 20 weeks, female fetuses already have all the eggs they will ever have in their ovaries — approximately 6 to 7 million, a number that will diminish to about 1 to 2 million by the time she is born.

What the Anatomy Scan Examines — A Full Account

The sonographer follows a systematic protocol, examining each structure in turn. Here is what is being assessed, and why:

The brain: The cerebral ventricles (fluid-filled spaces within the brain) are measured — enlargement (ventriculomegaly) can indicate various conditions. The cerebellum (the structure at the back of the brain responsible for coordination) is examined and measured. The corpus callosum (the bridge connecting the two hemispheres) is assessed. The fetal spine is scanned for any gaps or irregularities that might suggest spina bifida.

The face: The profile view shows the nasal bone (absent or small in some chromosomal conditions) and the position of the forehead, nose, lips, and chin. Cleft lip — a separation in the upper lip — can usually be identified at this scan. Cleft palate alone (without cleft lip) is much harder to see on ultrasound.

The heart: The four-chamber view of the heart is the most important cardiac assessment at this stage. The two atria and two ventricles should be approximately equal in size. The outflow tracts — the great vessels leaving the heart — are examined to detect transposition of the great arteries and other major cardiac abnormalities. Congenital heart disease affects approximately 8 in every 1,000 births; the anatomy scan detects the majority of significant abnormalities.

The abdomen: The position and appearance of the stomach (it should contain swallowed amniotic fluid, appearing as a dark bubble), the abdominal wall (to exclude gastroschisis — where intestines herniate outside the abdominal wall — or omphalocele), and the cord insertion point.

The kidneys and bladder: Both kidneys should be present and symmetrical. The bladder should contain urine (it empties every 20 to 30 minutes in utero). The renal pelvis diameter is measured — mild dilatation (pyelectasis) is common and usually resolves but warrants monitoring.

The limbs: All four limbs, with their long bones (femur, humerus, tibia, radius, etc.) measured and compared to gestational age norms. The hands and feet are examined; the position of the feet is checked for talipes (clubfoot).

The placenta: Location, appearance, and the position of the cord insertion. The most important finding is whether the placenta is covering the cervical os (placenta praevia) — if found at 20 weeks, a follow-up scan at 32 weeks is arranged, as most low-lying placentas migrate away from the os as the uterus grows.

Amniotic fluid: The volume of fluid is assessed — too little (oligohydramnios) or too much (polyhydramnios) can indicate various conditions.

If Something Is Found on the Scan

If the sonographer identifies a finding, they will either explain it to you directly or ask you to speak with your obstetrician. Findings fall broadly into three categories:

Soft markers: Minor findings of uncertain significance — small things like a slightly echogenic bowel (bright bowel on ultrasound), a short nasal bone, or echogenic intracardiac focus (a bright spot in the heart). Individually, these are usually of no significance. In combination, or in conjunction with a high-risk NT result or NIPT, they carry more weight. Your doctor will explain the clinical relevance of any soft marker found.

Significant findings requiring further assessment: Larger NT at this stage, ventriculomegaly, cardiac abnormalities, renal anomalies, skeletal abnormalities. These will prompt a referral to a fetal medicine specialist, detailed echocardiogram, and often a discussion about invasive testing.

Incidental findings unrelated to the baby: Ovarian cysts, uterine fibroids, low-lying placenta — all common findings that your doctor will explain and manage appropriately.

✍ My NOTE

When a finding is made on the anatomy scan, the next 24 hours are often among the most anxious of the entire pregnancy. The information arrives in a hospital setting, without preparation, and it is impossible to fully process in the moment. Please: if you receive an unexpected finding at your scan, make an appointment with your obstetrician as soon as possible — that day or the next. Write down your questions. Bring your partner. Do not spend the night on Google. What you find on Google will frighten you far more than the clinical reality usually warrants.

WEEKS 23–27

Viability and Vitality

Week 24 carries a weight that other weeks do not. It is the week of viability — the gestational age at which, with the best available neonatal care, survival outside the womb becomes possible. Not guaranteed; not without significant medical intervention and risk; but possible.

Obstetricians do not often say this out loud to patients, but reaching 24 weeks feels different from the inside of the profession too. Before 24 weeks, fetal loss — however devastating — is classified as a miscarriage and is managed primarily as a pregnancy loss. From 24 weeks, it becomes a preterm birth, and a neonatal team is involved. The medicine changes. The language changes. The possibilities change.

Your baby is still small — about 600 to 700 grams at 24 weeks — and her lungs are still immature. But she is developing with extraordinary speed.

♥ YOUR BABY RIGHT NOW

Weeks 24–27: 600–900 grams — the size of a small papaya or ear of corn

Your baby's face is fully formed and recognisably individual — if you could see her right now, you would know her when she is placed in your arms after birth. Her eyes are beginning to open. She has eyelashes. She is developing a sleep-wake cycle that you will begin to recognise as a pattern of activity and quiet. Her brain is developing its characteristic folds (gyri and sulci) — the cortical folding that massively increases the surface area of the brain and underlies higher cognitive function. Her lungs are producing surfactant, the critical substance that will allow her alveoli to inflate at birth rather than collapsing back. She responds to sound — startle responses to loud noises are now measurable. She responds to your touch — when you press gently on your abdomen, she may press back.

The Glucose Tolerance Test

Between 24 and 28 weeks, every pregnant woman should be tested for gestational diabetes mellitus (GDM). In India, this is not a recommendation to be skipped. Indian women have one of the highest global rates of GDM — estimates range from 10 to 25% in various Indian studies, compared with the global average of approximately 14%. The reason is our genetic predisposition to insulin resistance, which is pronounced in South Asian populations and is compounded by increasingly sedentary lifestyles and diet patterns.

The test itself — the 75-gram oral glucose tolerance test (OGTT) — requires you to come fasting (no food or drink except water for at least 8 hours). A fasting blood glucose is taken. You then drink a glucose solution containing 75 grams of glucose — it is very sweet, and some women find the taste nauseating. Blood is taken again at one hour and at two hours. Do not walk, exercise, or eat during the waiting period.

According to FOGSI (following IADPSG criteria), GDM is diagnosed if any one of the following is met: fasting glucose ≥92 mg/dL (5.1 mmol/L); one-hour glucose ≥180 mg/dL (10.0 mmol/L); two-hour glucose ≥153 mg/dL (8.5 mmol/L).

If You Are Diagnosed with GDM

A GDM diagnosis produces a particular kind of anxiety — the sense of having "failed" a test, of the pregnancy suddenly becoming complicated, of worry for the baby. I want to reframe this for you.

Gestational diabetes is extremely common. It is manageable. In the majority of cases, it is managed successfully with diet and exercise modifications alone. Your outcomes — for you and your baby — with well-managed GDM are excellent.

The immediate steps after a GDM diagnosis: A referral to a dietitian, ideally within a week. A blood glucose monitor and instruction on self-monitoring. Target blood glucose levels to aim for: fasting below 95 mg/dL (5.3 mmol/L), one hour after meals below 140 mg/dL (7.8 mmol/L), two hours after meals below 120 mg/dL (6.7 mmol/L). A schedule of closer antenatal monitoring, including growth scans.

If dietary management is not sufficient to maintain target levels within one to two weeks, medication is started. Insulin injections are the gold standard — they do not cross the placenta, are dose-adjustable, and have the longest safety record. Metformin tablets are used in many Indian centres as an alternative or adjunct, though it does cross the placenta (the available evidence is reassuring, but women should be aware of this and make an informed decision).

THE SCIENCE BEHIND IT

Why GDM Matters for Your Baby

When your blood sugar is elevated, glucose crosses the placenta freely and reaches the baby. Your baby's pancreas responds by producing more insulin — fetal insulin acts as a growth hormone, causing accelerated growth particularly in the abdomen (the Pedersen hypothesis). This is why babies of women with uncontrolled GDM can be very large (macrosomic).

The risks of poorly controlled GDM for the baby:

- Macrosomia (birth weight >4 kg) — increases risk of birth injury, shoulder dystocia
- Neonatal hypoglycaemia — when the umbilical cord is cut, the glucose supply stops, but the baby's insulin level remains high
- Stillbirth — the risk increases in poorly controlled GDM, particularly at and after term
- Increased caesarean section rate
- Long-term risk of obesity and type 2 diabetes for the child

The risks for you:

- Pre-eclampsia (2-4x increased risk)
- Caesarean section
- 50% lifetime risk of developing type 2 diabetes — a blood sugar test at 6-12 weeks postpartum and annual screening thereafter are essential

Your Growing Bump — Practical Realities

Backache

Lower back pain affects approximately 50 to 70% of pregnant women, and it commonly begins in the second trimester. The causes are multiple: the shifting centre of gravity as the bump grows (which causes increased lumbar lordosis — the exaggerated inward curve of the lower spine); the effect of the hormone relaxin, which loosens ligaments throughout the body in preparation for birth (helpful for the pelvis, less helpful for the spine); the growing uterus putting pressure on muscles and nerves; and, in many women, pre-existing postural issues that pregnancy simply makes more visible.

Pelvic girdle pain (PGP) — pain at the pubic symphysis and/or sacroiliac joints — is a related but distinct condition affecting approximately 20% of pregnant women. It can range from mild discomfort to severe disability that makes walking, climbing stairs, and turning in bed extremely difficult.

Management: Prenatal physiotherapy is the most evidence-based treatment and is genuinely helpful. A physiotherapist experienced in pregnancy will teach you core stabilisation exercises, posture correction, and movement strategies. Pelvic support belts can provide significant relief. Warm compresses, gentle pregnancy yoga, swimming, and sleeping with a pillow between your knees all help. Paracetamol is safe. NSAIDs (ibuprofen, diclofenac) should be avoided from 20 weeks onwards.

Heartburn

Gastro-oesophageal reflux — the burning sensation in the chest and throat that most people know as heartburn — affects up to 80% of pregnant women. It is caused by two things: progesterone relaxing the lower oesophageal sphincter (the valve between the oesophagus and stomach), allowing stomach acid to reflux upward; and the growing uterus physically compressing the stomach, pushing its contents upward.

Management: Eat small, frequent meals rather than large ones. Do not lie down for at least two hours after eating. Sleep with the head and upper body slightly elevated (extra pillows, or tilt the head of the bed). Avoid spicy, fatty, and acidic foods. Avoid large amounts of tea and coffee. Antacids (calcium carbonate preparations like Digene or Eno) are safe and often very effective. If antacids are not sufficient, your doctor can prescribe ranitidine (now with limitations due to NDMA concerns), famotidine, or omeprazole — all are considered safe in pregnancy when clinically indicated.

Varicose Veins and Haemorrhoids

Varicose veins — enlarged, twisted veins visible just below the skin surface, most commonly in the legs — affect approximately 40% of pregnant women. They are caused by the increased blood volume of pregnancy, the pressure of the uterus on the pelvic veins, and the softening effect of progesterone on vein walls. They are usually more unsightly than dangerous, though they can be uncomfortable and occasionally painful.

Prevention and management: Graduated compression stockings (worn from morning — before you get up — until bedtime), regular walking, elevating the legs when possible, and avoiding prolonged standing. Most varicosities improve after delivery.

Haemorrhoids (piles) — varicose veins of the anal canal — are another manifestation of the same process, compounded by the pressure of the uterus on pelvic veins and the constipation that many pregnant women experience. They affect approximately 25 to 35% of pregnant women. Management: stool softeners to prevent straining (lactulose, macrogol), topical creams (hydrocortisone preparations — brief use only), sitz baths, adequate hydration and fibre intake. Most improve dramatically after delivery.

Stretch Marks

Striae gravidarum — stretch marks — appear on the abdomen, breasts, thighs, and buttocks of approximately 50 to 90% of pregnant women. They are pink or reddish lines during pregnancy, fading to silver or white after delivery. They are caused by the rapid stretching of skin and the resulting disruption of collagen fibres in the dermis.

The honest truth about prevention: genetics plays the largest role in who gets stretch marks, and there is no cream or oil that has been proven in high-quality clinical trials to prevent them. Moisturising the skin regularly (coconut oil, almond oil, cocoa butter — whichever you prefer) can reduce the itching that often accompanies the stretching. Some women find regular massage helpful for comfort. But if you are going to get stretch marks — and many women are — no topical product will fully prevent them.

They are also, ultimately, the marks of a body that grew a human being. They deserve some respect.

" Ananya's Second Trimester

"Everyone keeps touching my stomach," Ananya said, at her 22-week appointment. "My mother-in-law, my colleagues, the aunty next door who I barely know. I did not consent to this." She looked partly amused, partly genuinely unsettled. "Is there a polite way to stop it?" I told her: yes. The polite way is to say, with a smile, "I would rather you didn't, thank you." This is a complete sentence. It requires no further explanation. Your body does not become public property because you are pregnant, and you are not obligated to tolerate uninvited touching simply because the person touching you is enthusiastic about your pregnancy.

WEEKS 24–27

Preparing Inside and Out

As the second trimester draws to a close, you may find your thoughts turning increasingly to the practicalities of what comes next. The third trimester — the final stretch — begins at week 28, and with it comes closer monitoring, the glucose test, the anti-D injection if you are Rh-negative, and the growing physical reality of a baby who is running out of room.

You may also be experiencing the very human phenomenon of beginning to mentally prepare for birth — reading, asking questions, attending antenatal classes, processing the birth stories of friends and family with a new intensity of interest.

Antenatal classes: These are worth attending, particularly for first-time parents. A good antenatal class — run by a trained midwife, physiotherapist, or obstetric nurse — will cover the stages of labour, pain relief options, what to expect in hospital, breastfeeding basics, and newborn care. It will also give you a room full of people in exactly the same stage of pregnancy as you, which has its own particular comfort.

If formal classes are not available to you, ask your doctor or midwife to walk you through the labour process. Read this book's chapters on birth. Watch evidence-based videos (organisations like Tommy's in the UK and FOGSI in India provide reliable online content). The more you know about what to expect, the less frightening the unknown becomes.

✔ WHAT TO DO THIS WEEK

✔ Have the 75g OGTT for gestational diabetes (24-28 weeks)

✔ Anti-D injection at 28 weeks if you are Rh negative

✔ Haemoglobin recheck — anaemia often worsens in the second trimester as blood volume expands

✔ Start monitoring fetal movements — you should feel distinct movements every day from 24 weeks

✔ Attend an antenatal class if available

✔ Begin to plan your hospital bag (see list in the appendix)

✔ Discuss your birth preferences with your doctor

✔ Begin sleeping on your left side — reduces pressure on the vena cava

✔ Review your workplace situation — maternity leave planning

✔ Sign up for a breastfeeding class or read the breastfeeding chapter of this book

4

The Third Trimester

Weeks 28 to 40: Almost There

You are in the home straight. Your baby is gaining weight rapidly and filling your uterus. Your body is beginning its long, slow preparation for birth. And you may find that the third trimester has a particular quality — a mixture of physical discomfort, practical urgency, and a growing emotional intensity that is unlike anything in the earlier months.

This is also the trimester when the reality of what is coming becomes undeniable. In the first trimester, birth was an abstract distant event. In the second, it was on the horizon. Now it is close. And whether your primary feeling is excited, terrified, or — most honestly — both simultaneously, this chapter will walk you through every week of it.

WEEKS 28–31

The Home Straight Begins

At 28 weeks, antenatal care intensifies. Visits that were monthly become fortnightly. Blood tests are repeated. The glucose test (if not already done) happens now. For women who are Rh negative, an anti-D immunoglobulin injection is given at 28 weeks and again at 34 weeks (or at delivery).

These changes are not incidental. The third trimester is when several significant pregnancy complications — pre-eclampsia, fetal growth restriction, gestational diabetes complications, placental issues — tend to present. The closer monitoring is specifically designed to catch these early.

♥ YOUR BABY RIGHT NOW

Weeks 28–31: 1.0–1.8 kg — the size of an aubergine or small cabbage

Your baby is gaining approximately 200 grams per week now. His brain is in its most rapid period of development: the cortex — the outer layer responsible for thought, language, and consciousness — is expanding dramatically, developing the characteristic folds and creases that distinguish a mature human brain from a smooth, early fetal one. He opens and closes his eyes. He has REM sleep — the rapid-eye-movement stage associated with dreaming in adults. He responds to pain and has a well-developed pain reflex. His immune system is receiving a transfusion of your antibodies through the placenta — protection against infections that will last for his first months of life. A baby born at 28 weeks today, in a well-equipped neonatal unit, has approximately an 85 to 90% chance of survival.

Fetal Movements: Your Most Important Daily Task

From 28 weeks onwards, monitoring your baby's movements every day is one of the most important things you can do for her safety. I want to be direct about this, because the message sometimes gets diluted: a significant reduction in fetal movements can be an early warning sign of fetal compromise. Acting on it promptly can save your baby's life.

The key word is "your." You know your baby's pattern better than any monitor, any scan, or any statistical average. Some babies are very active; some are naturally quieter. You have been feeling movements for weeks. You know what normal feels like for your baby specifically.

What you are watching for is a change from your baby's normal pattern. A day when she seems unusually still. A morning when the movements that usually wake you have not come. If you notice this, do not wait and see. Do not drink cold water and lie on your side for 20 minutes and decide it was nothing. Call your doctor or go to the maternity unit. Have the baby assessed. If everything is fine — and usually it is — you will go home reassured. But occasionally it is not fine, and the fact that you came in when you did made the difference.

REDUCED FETAL MOVEMENTS — ACT TODAY, NOT TOMORROW

From 28 weeks, you should feel your baby move every day. If you notice:

- Fewer movements than usual for your baby
- No movements for 2 hours after eating and lying on your left side
- Movements that feel different — weaker, less vigorous than usual

Then: call your doctor or go to the maternity unit immediately.

Do NOT: wait until tomorrow. Be reassured by one glass of cold water. Assume the baby is sleeping. Feel embarrassed about calling.

There is no such thing as "the baby is running out of space and moving less." Normal babies move every day until birth. A reduction is always worth investigating.

Third-Trimester Antenatal Visits

From 28 weeks, visits become fortnightly (every two weeks) and then, from 36 weeks, weekly. At each visit, your doctor will measure your blood pressure, test your urine for protein (screening for pre-eclampsia), check your weight, feel your abdomen to assess fundal height and fetal position, and listen to the fetal heart.

Growth scans: Women with risk factors for fetal growth restriction (previous small baby, hypertension, smoking, multiple pregnancy, chronic conditions) will be scheduled for serial growth scans — typically at 28, 32, and 36 weeks. At each scan, the estimated fetal weight (EFW) is plotted on a growth chart. What matters is not just the weight at a single point but the pattern of growth over time. A baby whose EFW crosses centile lines downward — growing more slowly than expected — raises concern for placental insufficiency, even if the absolute weight is within normal range.

Doppler assessment: If fetal growth restriction is suspected, Doppler ultrasound assesses blood flow in the umbilical artery (measuring placental resistance) and the middle cerebral artery (measuring whether the brain is compensating by "stealing" blood from other organs). Reduced or absent end-diastolic flow in the umbilical artery is a serious finding that significantly changes management.

WEEKS 32–36

The Final Preparations

These weeks have a particular quality. Your baby is gaining weight rapidly and beginning to look like the baby you will meet. Your body is making increasingly noticeable preparations for birth. And practically, you have approximately four to eight weeks to get ready — for the hospital, for the home, for the completely new reality of your life after birth.

♥ YOUR BABY RIGHT NOW

Weeks 32–36: 1.8–2.7 kg — the size of a small melon or large coconut

Your baby's face has subcutaneous fat now — it is rounded, soft-looking, the face you will recognise immediately when you see it. His lungs are producing surfactant in increasing quantities; a baby born after 34 weeks rarely needs respiratory support. He is practising breathing, hiccupping regularly (those rhythmic, repetitive jerks you feel are hiccups — entirely normal), and swallowing amniotic fluid at a rate of up to 700 mL per day. His fingernails and toenails have grown to the ends of his fingers and toes. His skull bones are firm but not yet fused — they will overlap during birth (moulding) to allow passage through the birth canal, and return to their normal shape within a few days after birth.

The Baby's Position

From around 34 weeks, fetal position becomes clinically important. The optimal position for birth is cephalic — head down, with the back of the baby's head facing the front of your abdomen (occiput anterior, or OA). This is also the most common position, because it represents the most efficient use of space in the uterus as the baby grows.

At 34 weeks, approximately 96% of babies are in cephalic presentation. At 36 weeks, the remaining 4% who are still breech are offered an External Cephalic Version (ECV) — a procedure performed in hospital under ultrasound guidance, in which a doctor applies firm pressure on the outside of the abdomen to manually turn the baby head-down. ECV is successful in approximately 50 to 60% of attempts, is safe (with appropriate fetal monitoring before and after), and significantly reduces the likelihood of caesarean section.

Another position worth understanding is occiput posterior (OP) — where the baby's head is down but its back is against your back rather than facing forward. This is also called "back to back" and often causes significant back labour — labour pain that is felt predominantly in the lower back rather than the abdomen. Most OP babies rotate during labour; some do not. Hands-and-knees positioning and rocking movements in labour can encourage rotation.

Preparing Your Hospital Bag

The hospital bag conversation provokes enormous anxiety — every list you find online is different, and every other mother you speak to has strong opinions. Here is a practical, reasonable list:

For You in Labour

- Your antenatal records (keep these accessible — many women carry them in their bag from 36 weeks)
- Your ID and insurance documents or government health scheme card
- A comfortable, loose nightgown or long top — something you do not mind getting stained
- Your mobile phone and charger
- Lip balm — breathing through contractions is drying
- Snacks and drinks for your partner — they will be there a long time
- A list of your birth preferences
- Earphones and music or a meditation app if these help you relax

After Delivery

For You

- 3 to 4 comfortable loose nightgowns or kaftans (front-opening if you plan to breastfeed)
- High-waisted comfortable underwear — at least 5 pairs
- Maternity pads — thick, absorbent (not regular sanitary pads; postpartum bleeding is heavier)
- Nursing bras if breastfeeding — at least 2 or 3, sized for larger breasts than your current size
- Nipple cream (lanolin-based)
- Toiletries and personal care items
- Going-home outfit (loose, comfortable — you will still look 6 months pregnant for some weeks after birth)

For the Baby

- 3 to 4 newborn onesies or jhablas
- 2 to 3 warm layers (the hospital may be air-conditioned)
- Newborn nappies/diapers or cloth nappies
- A warm blanket
- Car seat if you are travelling home by car (required by law in many countries; safest practice everywhere)

✍ My NOTE

A note about the hospital bag: pack it by 36 weeks. Not because most first babies come before their due date (they usually do not), but because packing it means you have had a practical conversation with yourself and your partner about what you need, where you are going, who is driving, and what the plan is. That conversation is worth more than the bag.

WEEKS 37–40

Any Day Now

"Full term" begins at 37 weeks. Your baby is considered mature. Her lungs, her brain, her liver — all the systems that need to function independently at birth — are ready. The remaining weeks are finishing touches: weight gain, further fat deposition, the final maturation of the immune system, and the transfer of your antibodies.

These final weeks have a quality of suspended time. You are ready. Your body is ready. And yet the baby arrives on her own schedule, which frequently ignores yours. First babies in particular are notoriously late — the average gestational age at first birth is approximately 40 weeks and 3 days. This is normal. It is also, by week 40, extremely frustrating.

♥ YOUR BABY RIGHT NOW

Weeks 38–40: 3.0–3.5 kg — ready for the world

Your baby has now received the maximum transfer of your antibodies — she is as immunologically equipped as she can be at birth. Her skull plates are mobile and will overlap during delivery, allowing her head to temporarily reshape to fit the birth canal (moulding) — this is normal and resolves within days. She has well-developed reflexes: sucking, rooting (turning toward touch on the cheek), grasping, and startle. She can hear, see (though her vision is initially blurred and limited to about 25-30 cm), smell, and taste. She knows your voice. She has been hearing it her entire conscious existence. She is ready. And in some deep, cellular, unknowable way — you are ready too.

Signs of Labour: The Complete Guide

The final weeks of pregnancy are accompanied by a great deal of uncertainty about when labour will begin. Here is a comprehensive guide to the signs — and what they mean.

Braxton-Hicks Contractions vs True Labour

Braxton-Hicks contractions — the irregular tightenings of the uterus that have been occurring since as early as the second trimester but become more noticeable in the third — intensify significantly in the final weeks. They can be uncomfortable and can closely mimic early labour contractions. The key differences:

Braxton-Hicks: Irregular (no consistent pattern of frequency). Do not increase in intensity over time. Often ease or stop when you change position, walk around, or drink water. Felt mainly in the front of the abdomen. Not accompanied by cervical change.

True labour contractions: Regular (gradually becoming more frequent). Progressive (becoming longer, stronger, and closer together over time). Do not ease with position change or walking — in fact, walking may intensify them. Often felt starting in the lower back and radiating around to the front. Accompanied by progressive cervical effacement and dilation.

The Show

The "show" — or mucous plug — is a blob of thick, jelly-like mucus that has sealed the cervical canal throughout the pregnancy, acting as a protective barrier. As the cervix begins to soften and efface (thin out) in the days or weeks before labour, this plug is released. It may come as one piece or in smaller amounts over several days. It is often tinged pink or brown from small amounts of blood as the cervix's tiny blood vessels stretch.

The show is a sign that your cervix is beginning to prepare for labour. Labour may follow within hours, or it may be several days or even a week away. If the show is accompanied by heavy bleeding or regular contractions, contact your doctor.

Waters Breaking

Rupture of the amniotic membranes — "waters breaking" — occurs in approximately 10 to 15% of labours before contractions begin. It may be a dramatic gush (as in films, though usually less dramatic) or a continuous small trickle that some women mistake for urinary leakage.

How to tell the difference between amniotic fluid and urine: Amniotic fluid is clear or slightly yellow, odourless, and does not stop when you try to stop it (unlike urine). Wear a pad; lie down for 30 minutes, then stand up — if you feel a fresh gush or continuing trickle, your waters have broken.

If you believe your waters have broken: call your maternity unit or doctor, regardless of whether contractions have started. Once the amniotic sac is ruptured, the baby's protective barrier is gone and the risk of infection (chorioamnionitis) increases with time. Most units advise coming in for assessment within a few hours, and recommend delivery within 12 to 24 hours if contractions do not begin spontaneously.

♡ WHAT YOU MIGHT BE FEELING

- Pelvic pressure and heaviness as the baby's head descends into the pelvis
- Increased urinary frequency as the baby's head presses on the bladder
- "Lightening" — the bump may appear to sit lower, and you can breathe more easily as the baby drops out of the ribcage
- Disrupted sleep — between needing to urinate, discomfort finding a position, and an active mind, deep sleep becomes difficult
- Nesting instinct — a sudden, powerful urge to prepare, organise, clean. Listen to it. Do not overdo it.
- Increasing anxiety about birth — this is universal. Talk about it with your doctor.
- Braxton-Hicks contractions becoming stronger and more frequent
- Emotional readiness — a deep knowledge that you are as prepared as you will ever be

✔ WHAT TO DO THIS WEEK

✔ Pack your hospital bag — by 36 weeks

✔ Discuss induction of labour with your doctor — offered to most women by 41-42 weeks

✔ Attend your weekly appointments from 36 weeks

✔ GBS swab at 35-37 weeks (in units that screen for Group B Streptococcus)

✔ Tdap vaccine if not yet given this pregnancy

✔ Discuss birth preferences with your doctor — write a simple plan

✔ Arrange post-delivery support: who will help you at home in the first weeks?

✔ Prepare the baby's space at home

✔ Confirm your transport plan to hospital

✔ Rest. Sleep when you can. You are about to need your reserves.

" Meena's Last Four Weeks

"I am enormous," Meena said at her 38-week appointment, settling into the chair with the specific care of a woman whose every movement requires planning. "My mother has moved in. My mother-in-law has opinions about my mother moving in. My husband is pretending not to notice the tension. I have not slept in three weeks. And my ankles — look at them." I looked. They were, indeed, impressive. I told her what I tell every woman in those final weeks: every day of discomfort is a day of your baby growing stronger. Every sleepless night is your body practising for what comes next. It does not make the discomfort easier — but it gives it meaning. Meena's daughter arrived at 39+4, eight pounds exactly, spectacularly healthy. The ankles returned to normal within a week.

5

Birth

The Day That Changes Everything

There is no single way to give birth. There is no correct way, no superior way, no way that makes you more or less of a mother. There is only your birth — shaped by your body, your baby, your circumstances, and the decisions you make together with your medical team on the day.

What I can give you is knowledge. Knowledge of what labour feels like from the inside — the physical sensations, the emotional waves, the moments of doubt and the moments of extraordinary power. Knowledge of what your body is doing at each stage and why. Knowledge of your options, so that when choices need to be made — and some choices will need to be made in the middle of it, without time to research — you have a foundation.

I have stood beside thousands of women in labour. What I have learned, above everything, is this: women are stronger than they know. The body is smarter than it looks from the outside. And birth, for all its difficulty, is one of the most profound experiences that human life offers.

How Labour Begins

Labour is not switched on by a single event. It is initiated by a complex cascade of hormonal signals involving the baby, the placenta, and the mother — a conversation between three parties that has been building gradually for weeks before you notice anything at all.

The baby plays an active role in initiating labour. As the fetal lungs mature, they begin producing a protein called surfactant protein A, which triggers an inflammatory cascade in the uterus that promotes prostaglandin production. Cortisol produced by the fetal adrenal glands also rises steadily in the final weeks, contributing to uterine activation. This is why premature rupture of membranes and preterm labour are more common in conditions of fetal stress — the baby's physiology is accelerating the process.

From the mother's side, oxytocin receptors in the uterus proliferate dramatically in the final weeks of pregnancy, making the uterus increasingly sensitive to the oxytocin already circulating. Prostaglandins produced locally in the cervix cause it to soften, efface (thin), and dilate. Relaxin from the placenta loosens the ligaments of the pelvic girdle, creating flexibility for the baby's passage.

The result of all of this preparation is a uterus poised and ready — waiting for the final trigger, which when it comes, sets off a self-amplifying cycle of contractions that grows progressively stronger until the baby is born.

The First Stage of Labour

The Latent Phase

The latent phase is early labour — the period from the onset of regular contractions to approximately 5 to 6 centimetres of cervical dilation. It is the longest phase of labour, particularly for first-time mothers, and it is often the most frustrating.

Contractions during the latent phase are usually irregular — coming every 5 to 20 minutes, lasting 30 to 45 seconds, and of moderate intensity. They are uncomfortable but not typically the overwhelming, all-consuming contractions of active labour. Many women can talk through them. Many continue normal activities between them.

The latent phase can last anywhere from a few hours to more than 24 hours in first-time mothers. It does not follow a timetable. It cannot be hurried. And it is almost always best managed at home.

At home during the latent phase:

- Rest as much as possible — if contractions begin at night, try to sleep between them. The energy you preserve now will be needed later.

- Eat light, easily digestible food if you can — toast, banana, yoghurt. You may not want to eat in active labour.
- Stay hydrated — drink water regularly throughout.
- Move in ways that feel comfortable — walking, rocking, swaying on a birth ball, warm bath or shower.
- Time your contractions — use a contraction timer app. Note when they become regular (every 5 minutes), lasting at least 1 minute, for at least 1 hour. This is the general guideline for when to go to hospital (the "5-1-1 rule").
- Have your partner or support person with you.

✍ My NOTE

The most common mistake in early labour is going to hospital too soon. I understand the impulse — when contractions begin, the instinct is to get to the place where the baby will be born as quickly as possible. But arriving at hospital at 2 centimetres dilation means waiting in a clinical environment, often on a foetal monitor, in a room that is not yours, for something that may be many hours away. Women who labour at home in the early phase tend to cope better, use less pain relief, and have fewer interventions. Stay home until contractions are strong, regular, and 5 minutes apart. Then come.

The Active Phase

Active labour begins at approximately 5 to 6 centimetres of dilation. The contractions are now unmistakable: strong, long (60 seconds or more), regular (every 3 to 4 minutes), and requiring your full attention. You can no longer talk through them. They demand that you stop, focus, breathe, and ride them.

Progress in active labour is typically faster than in the latent phase: approximately 0.5 to 1 centimetre per hour in first-time mothers, somewhat faster in subsequent labours. At this rate, active labour from 5 to 10 centimetres takes roughly 5 to 10 hours for first-time mothers, though there is enormous individual variation.

The cervix does not dilate at a perfectly linear rate. It may stay at 6 centimetres for what feels like a very long time and then open rapidly. This is normal. The cervix dilates in surges, not smoothly. A single vaginal examination showing "no progress" does not mean labour has stopped.

Transition

Transition is the period between the end of the first stage (when the cervix is nearly fully dilated, usually 8 to 10 centimetres) and the beginning of the second stage. It is typically the most intense part of labour, and mercifully, it is also usually the shortest.

Contractions during transition are very strong and may come in rapid succession with only brief intervals between them. Many women feel overwhelmed, shaky, nauseous, or suddenly despairing — "I cannot do this" is one of the most commonly reported thoughts during transition. This is not weakness. This is transition. The fact that you feel this way is often a sign that you are nearly there. The baby is coming.

What helps in transition: the continuous presence of a trusted support person; a calm, steady voice saying that you are doing well and that this is almost over; short, focused breathing; and the knowledge that this intensity is temporary — transition rarely lasts more than 30 to 60 minutes.

The Second Stage: Pushing and Birth

The second stage begins when the cervix reaches 10 centimetres — full dilation — and ends with the birth of your baby. It is announced by a change in the sensation of contractions: instead of (or in addition to) the wave of pain, you may feel a powerful, involuntary urge to push — a bearing-down sensation that is sometimes described as resembling an overwhelming need to have a bowel movement. This is the Ferguson reflex, triggered by the baby's presenting part pressing on stretch receptors in the pelvic floor.

With an epidural, this urge may be blunted or absent. This is why, with an epidural in place, the second stage is often managed with delayed pushing — waiting an hour after full dilation before beginning to push, allowing the baby time to descend passively. Studies show this "labouring down" approach reduces the pushing time without worsening outcomes.

Pushing technique: At the peak of a contraction, take a breath, hold it, and push downward with your pelvic floor — as if trying to have a bowel movement. Hold for as long as you can (ideally 6 to 8 seconds), then breathe, then push again. Most contractions allow for 2 to 3 pushes. Between contractions, rest completely.

Pushing with epidural: If you cannot feel the contraction, your midwife or nurse will guide you — "push now" — based on the CTG trace showing the contraction peak.

The length of the second stage varies enormously. For first-time mothers without an epidural, up to 2 hours is considered within normal range; with an epidural, up to 3 hours. For subsequent births, the second stage is typically much shorter — often 10 to 30 minutes.

Crowning and Delivery

Crowning is the moment when the widest diameter of the baby's head stretches the vaginal opening and can be seen between pushes as well as during them. It is accompanied by a burning, stretching sensation that many women describe as a "ring of fire" — intense but brief, lasting only a few pushes.

Your midwife or doctor will guide you at this point: usually asking you to stop pushing and to pant — short, light breaths — while they support the perineum and allow the baby's head to emerge slowly and gently. This controlled delivery of the head reduces the risk of severe perineal tearing.

With the next push or two, the baby's head is delivered. The midwife or doctor checks for the umbilical cord around the neck (a nuchal cord) — present in approximately 25% of births and usually easily managed. The baby's shoulders follow, one at a time, and then with a rush — the body.

♥ YOUR BABY RIGHT NOW

The Moment of Birth

Your baby has spent his entire existence in fluid, in warmth, in the rhythmic sounds of your heartbeat. In the seconds of birth, everything changes simultaneously: he moves from warm water to cool air, from muffled sounds to clear ones, from the nutrition of the umbilical cord to the independent task of breathing. His first breath inflates lungs that have never been inflated. The dramatic pressure changes force fluid out of the alveoli. He cries — and that cry is the sound of lungs working, of a cardiovascular system re-routing, of a new person announcing himself to the world. Place him on your chest. He knows your heartbeat. He knows your voice. He has been waiting to meet you.

The Third Stage: Delivering the Placenta

After your baby is born, the uterus continues to contract. These contractions separate the placenta from the uterine wall and deliver it, usually within 5 to 30 minutes of the baby's birth.

Active management of the third stage — the standard of care in most hospitals — involves an injection of oxytocin (10 IU intramuscularly) given in your thigh as the baby is born or immediately after, followed by controlled cord traction (gentle, steady pulling on the umbilical cord) once signs of placental separation are present. This approach, recommended by WHO and FOGSI, reduces the risk of postpartum haemorrhage by approximately 50%.

Delayed cord clamping — waiting at least 1 to 3 minutes before cutting the cord — is now recommended as standard practice. In the first minutes after birth, the placenta continues to pump blood into the baby through the cord, delivering 80 to 100 mL of additional blood. This blood is rich in iron, stem cells, and immune factors. Delayed cord clamping has been shown to reduce the risk of iron-deficiency anaemia in infancy, improve iron stores, and may have neurological benefits. It is compatible with active management of the third stage.

Pain Relief: A Guide

Pain in labour is real, intense, and variable. It is caused by uterine contractions (ischaemic pain — the muscle working hard against resistance), cervical dilation (stretching and pressure pain), and the descent and delivery of the baby through the pelvis (pressure and stretch). The experience of labour pain is highly individual: the same physiological event can be very differently experienced by different women, and by the same woman in different labours.

You have the right to as much pain relief as you need. You also have the right to manage labour without pharmacological pain relief if that is your choice. There is no virtue in suffering, but there is also no shame in wanting an unmedicated birth. The goal is an informed choice, made freely, by you.

Non-Pharmacological Pain Relief

Continuous support — the single most evidence-based intervention for improving labour outcomes. A Cochrane review of over 15,000 women found that continuous one-to-one support throughout labour (from a doula, partner, or dedicated midwife) reduced caesarean section rates, reduced the need for pain medication, shortened labour, and improved women's satisfaction with the birth experience. This is not a complementary add-on. It is medicine, and it should be treated as such.

Water immersion — a warm bath or shower in early to active labour significantly reduces pain, promotes relaxation, and reduces anxiety. Many women find the transition from land to water provides immediate, dramatic relief. Most hospitals now have shower facilities in labour rooms; some have birthing pools. Being in water does not increase infection risk when membranes are intact.

Movement and positioning — upright positions (walking, standing, swaying, kneeling, all-fours) use gravity to promote fetal descent, open the pelvic diameter, and often reduce back labour pain. Lying flat on your back is generally the least comfortable and least efficient position for labour, despite being the position most associated with birth in popular imagery (this is because it is convenient for medical attendants, not because it is optimal for you).

Heat — a heat pack on the lower back or abdomen provides genuine comfort during contractions. Hot water bottles, heat pads, and warm towels are all options. Not too hot — your skin is sensitive in labour.

Breathing — slow, rhythmic breathing during contractions is not merely a distraction technique. It activates the parasympathetic nervous system, reduces adrenaline, and genuinely modulates the pain experience. The simplest technique: breathe in slowly for a count of 4, out for a count of 6 to 8. Focus on the out-breath.

TENS (Transcutaneous Electrical Nerve Stimulation) — small electrical pulses applied to the lower back via electrode pads. Moderate evidence for effectiveness, particularly in early labour. Can be used at home. Has no side effects. The sensation takes some getting used to.

Pharmacological Pain Relief

Nitrous oxide (Entonox or "laughing gas") — inhaled through a mouthpiece at the onset of each contraction. It takes approximately 30 seconds to take effect, so you must begin inhaling as the contraction starts, before the peak. It provides moderate analgesia and significant anxiolysis (anxiety reduction). Its effects wear off within minutes of stopping. Some women find it excellent; others find it makes them feel nauseous or dissociated. It is safe for the baby.

Opioids — pethidine (meperidine) 50 to 100 mg intramuscularly, or morphine, provide moderate pain relief and sedation. They are useful in the latent phase when sleep is possible, or when other methods are insufficient and an epidural is not yet desired or available. The main limitation: if given within 4 hours of birth, opioids can cause neonatal respiratory depression. This is reversible with naloxone administered to the baby — but it is preferable to time opioid use so that the effect has worn off by delivery. They also cross to the baby in all doses and can cause initial drowsiness that may affect early breastfeeding.

Epidural analgesia — the gold standard for labour pain relief. A thin catheter is placed in the epidural space in the lower back under local anaesthesia. A continuous infusion of local anaesthetic (usually bupivacaine) with a small amount of opioid (fentanyl) provides near-complete pain relief for approximately 90% of women. Modern low-dose epidurals allow preservation of lower limb strength and sensation, enabling women to change position and sometimes to walk.

Common concerns about epidurals, answered honestly:

- "Does it increase my risk of caesarean?" — No. Multiple high-quality studies, including randomised controlled trials, have consistently shown that epidurals do not increase caesarean section rates.
- "Does it slow down labour?" — It may slightly prolong the second stage (by about 15 to 20 minutes on average). This is clinically managed by allowing adequate time for pushing.
- "Does it cause permanent back pain?" — No. This is one of the most persistent and thoroughly refuted myths in obstetrics. Post-epidural back pain is caused by the musculoskeletal strain of labour, not the epidural itself.
- "Is it bad for the baby?" — The baby receives very little of the medication (much less than with systemic opioids) because local anaesthetics do not cross the placenta efficiently. Epidurals are safe for the baby.
- "Can I request one at any point?" — Yes. There is no cervical dilation limit beyond which epidurals cannot be placed. You can request one at 2 cm or at 9 cm.

Caesarean Section: Understanding Your Options

A caesarean section is the delivery of a baby through a surgical incision in the abdomen and uterus. It is one of the most commonly performed surgical procedures in the world and, when performed for appropriate indications, is a lifesaving operation. In India, the caesarean rate is approximately 17% nationally – rising to 40 to 50% in some private sector hospitals.

Not all of these caesareans are medically necessary. This is a documented reality in Indian and global obstetric practice. Understanding why caesareans are performed helps you to be an informed participant in decisions about your own birth.

Emergency vs Planned Caesarean

A planned (elective) caesarean is scheduled in advance, usually from 39 weeks. Indications include: placenta praevia (placenta covering the cervix); breech presentation that cannot be or has not been corrected; certain maternal medical conditions; two or more previous caesarean sections; a previous classical (vertical) uterine incision.

An emergency caesarean is performed when an indication develops unexpectedly – during labour or in the antenatal period. Common indications: failure to progress in labour despite adequate contractions and appropriate time; fetal heart rate changes suggesting fetal distress that cannot be managed expectantly; cord prolapse (umbilical cord descending past the baby's presenting part); placental abruption; maternal haemorrhage.

Emergency caesareans are classified into four categories by urgency: Category 1 (immediate threat to life – performed within 30 minutes), Category 2 (maternal or fetal compromise, not immediately life-threatening – within 75 minutes), Category 3 (no immediate compromise, needs early delivery), and Category 4 (planned).

VBAC: Vaginal Birth After Caesarean

If you have had one previous caesarean section, you are likely a candidate for vaginal birth in your next pregnancy — this is called VBAC (Vaginal Birth After Caesarean). The success rate of VBAC in appropriately selected women is 60 to 80%. The risks and benefits of VBAC versus repeat elective caesarean (ERCS) need to be discussed with your obstetrician individually, but in general:

Advantages of VBAC: Shorter recovery, no surgical risks, ability to have more pregnancies without cumulative caesarean complications, better outcomes for the baby in terms of breathing difficulties and microbiome.

The main risk of VBAC: Uterine rupture — tearing of the previous scar during labour. This risk is approximately 0.5 to 0.7% — roughly 1 in 150 to 200 labours. Uterine rupture is a serious emergency but, with appropriate monitoring in a hospital setting, is almost always survivable for both mother and baby.

VBAC is not appropriate for everyone. Women with two or more previous caesareans, previous classical incision, previous uterine rupture, or this pregnancy's indication being the same as the previous caesarean are generally recommended to have a planned repeat caesarean.

✍ My NOTE

I am sometimes asked by women whether they can choose to have a caesarean without a medical indication. This is called caesarean on maternal request (CDMR). It is a conversation worth having with your doctor — understanding your specific risks and benefits, your previous experiences, and your values. I will never dismiss this request or make a woman feel judged for asking. But I will always ensure she has complete information first. Caesarean section is major surgery, and the risks — particularly for future pregnancies — accumulate with each one.

Your Birth Plan

A birth plan is a written summary of your preferences for labour and delivery, what you would like in an ideal scenario, and what matters most to you. It is not a contract or a guarantee. Birth, by its nature, does not always go according to plan. But the process of writing one forces important conversations and ensures that your medical team knows your priorities.

A useful birth plan covers: who you want present during labour and delivery; your preferences for pain relief (what you would like to try first, what you are open to, what you want to avoid if possible); your position preferences for pushing; your wishes regarding episiotomy; delayed cord clamping; immediate skin-to-skin contact; breastfeeding in the first hour; and what you would want if a caesarean becomes necessary.

Keep it brief — one page is ideal. Your midwife and doctor will not have time to read three pages during active labour. Bullet points, not paragraphs.

" Kavya's Birth

"My birth plan said: no epidural, stay mobile, minimal intervention," Kavya told me at her six-week postnatal check. She paused, then smiled. "By hour twelve I had the epidural, an oxytocin drip, and was very grateful for all of it." She had laboured for sixteen hours, progressed to nine centimetres, and then the baby's heart rate began showing patterns that concerned me. We discussed it honestly. She asked good questions. She understood what I was seeing. She agreed to the caesarean. Her son was born within twenty minutes, screaming, eight pounds and four ounces of indignant perfection. "I didn't get the birth I planned," she said. "I got him healthy. Which was the actual plan."

6

The Fourth Trimester

You, Your Baby, and the First Weeks

The fourth trimester is a term used to describe the first three months of your baby's life outside the womb. It acknowledges something that traditional maternity care has often overlooked: the transition from pregnancy to new parenthood is its own distinct phase, with its own challenges, its own developmental milestones, and its own need for support and understanding.

Your baby has arrived in the world. She is small, new, and completely dependent on you. Your body has just been through one of the most significant physical events of your entire life. Your hormones are in freefall. You are not sleeping. And yet the world — your in-laws, your colleagues, social media — is already asking about your baby's milestones and whether you have "got your body back."

Let me say this clearly: the fourth trimester is about you as much as your baby. It is about your recovery, your adjustment, your new identity. And it deserves the same attention and preparation as every other part of this journey.

Your Body in the First Hours

Immediately after birth — whether vaginal or by caesarean — the first priority is your safety and your baby's wellbeing. In the first hour or two (the "golden hour"), several things happen:

Your uterus begins to contract back down. The fundus (top of the uterus), which was at your navel at the time of delivery, descends over the following days and weeks as the uterus involutes — returning from its pregnant weight of approximately 1,000 grams to its non-pregnant weight of 50 to 80 grams. You will feel this involution as "afterpains" — uterine contractions that are often strongest during breastfeeding (because feeding triggers oxytocin, which contracts the uterus). Afterpains are typically stronger in second and subsequent pregnancies.

Vaginal bleeding (lochia) begins immediately after delivery and continues for 4 to 6 weeks. It changes in character over time: lochia rubra (bright red, first 3 to 4 days), lochia serosa (pinkish-brown, days 4 to 10), lochia alba (creamy white, days 10 to 28 or later). Heavier bleeding when you feed the baby, or when you stand up after lying down, is normal. Sudden heavy bleeding soaking more than one pad an hour, or passing large clots, warrants immediate attention.

Temperature regulation fluctuates dramatically in the first hours. You may feel intensely cold and shivery immediately after birth (a normal physiological response to the sudden hormonal and circulatory changes) and then become very warm. This is not infection. It is physiology.

Vaginal Birth Recovery

The perineum has done extraordinary work. Whether it tore spontaneously or was cut (episiotomy), and whether you had sutures or not, it needs time and attention to heal.

First-degree tears involve only the skin and mucous membrane of the vaginal opening. They may or may not be sutured and typically heal within 1 to 2 weeks.

Second-degree tears extend into the perineal muscles. They are sutured in layers under local anaesthesia and typically heal well within 2 to 4 weeks, though tenderness may persist longer.

Third and fourth-degree tears extend into the anal sphincter and, in fourth-degree tears, into the rectal mucosa. These are repaired in the operating theatre under spinal or general anaesthesia by a trained surgeon. They heal well when properly repaired, but require careful follow-up for months after delivery, as there is a risk of faecal incontinence or urgency if the sphincter repair breaks down.

Perineal Care at Home

- Ice packs wrapped in a cloth in the first 24 hours reduce swelling and provide significant pain relief.

- Sitz baths — sitting in a few inches of warm water for 15 to 20 minutes, two to three times daily — promote healing and provide comfort. A clean plastic tub placed in the bathroom is ideal; alternatively, a shallow bath.
- Pouring warm water over the perineum while urinating reduces the stinging discomfort of urine on healing skin.
- Paracetamol and ibuprofen (if not contraindicated) taken regularly, not just when pain becomes severe, are significantly more effective at managing perineal pain than taking them intermittently.
- Lignocaine (lidocaine) gel applied topically provides temporary surface anaesthesia and can be very helpful for the first week.
- Keep the area clean and dry. Shower daily. Pat dry rather than rub.
- Begin pelvic floor exercises within 24 hours of birth, even if this feels completely impossible. Even attempting the contraction, even if no movement is felt, begins the recovery process. Do them lying down at first if that is easier.

Caesarean Section Recovery

A caesarean section is major abdominal surgery. It involves incision through the abdominal skin, subcutaneous fat, fascia, and uterine wall — five or six separate layers. Recovery is correspondingly significant, and the culture that encourages women to be "up and about" quickly can sometimes cause more harm than good.

The First 24 to 48 Hours

You will have a urinary catheter in place for approximately 12 to 24 hours after surgery. An intravenous line provides fluids and medications. You will be given regular pain relief — typically paracetamol, ibuprofen (when tolerated), and a low-dose opioid for the first day or two. Take the pain relief regularly, on schedule. Do not wait until you are in significant pain to ask for medication.

You will be asked to get up and walk within 12 to 24 hours — this feels impossible but is genuinely important for preventing blood clots. The first time you get up, do so with support. Movement will become easier over the following days.

You will be given daily injections of low-molecular-weight heparin for 10 days after surgery (or 6 weeks if there are additional risk factors for thromboembolism) to prevent blood clots. You will also be given compression stockings to wear until you are fully mobile.

Going Home After Caesarean

Most women are discharged 3 to 4 days after an uncomplicated caesarean. At home:

- Keep the wound clean and dry. Pat dry gently after showering. Do not allow the wound to stay damp.
- Watch for signs of wound infection: increasing redness, warmth, swelling, discharge from the wound, fever, or increasing rather than decreasing pain. Any of these warrants a call to your doctor.
- Do not lift anything heavier than your baby for the first 4 to 6 weeks. This is not optional — lifting risks disrupting the healing of the internal uterine incision, which takes considerably longer to heal than the skin.
- Do not drive for 6 weeks, and only when you feel confident you could perform an emergency stop without hesitation or pain.
- Bathing (submerging the wound) should wait until the wound is completely closed — typically 3 to 4 weeks.
- You may notice numbness above the wound — this is caused by the incision cutting small sensory nerves and may persist for months. It usually resolves with time.

✍ **My NOTE**

Many women who have had a caesarean feel a complicated mix of emotions about it — relief that it is over, gratitude for the outcome, but sometimes grief, anger, or a sense of failure about not having had a vaginal birth. These feelings are legitimate and deserve to be acknowledged, not dismissed. If you find yourself struggling with how your birth went, please talk about it — with your doctor, your partner, or a counsellor. Processing a birth experience is important, however it went.

Breastfeeding: Everything You Need to Know

Breastfeeding is described as "natural" — and it is, in the sense that the biological capacity is built in. But it is also a learned skill, for both mother and baby, and like all learned skills, it requires practice, patience, and often support before it becomes comfortable.

The fact that many women struggle with breastfeeding is not a failure of nature. It is a consequence of living in a world where breastfeeding skills are no longer transmitted automatically through community and observation, where women often have their first breastfeeding experience alone in a hospital bed with a baby who has never eaten before, and where the support available is variable in quality and often insufficient in duration.

The First Hour: Skin to Skin

The single most powerful thing you can do for breastfeeding success is place your baby skin-to-skin on your chest in the first hour after birth — the "golden hour." Skin-to-skin contact triggers a cascade of responses in both you and your baby: your oxytocin rises (promoting bonding and milk production), your baby's rooting and sucking reflexes are activated, your baby's temperature and blood sugar are stabilised, and the sensory input of your heartbeat and smell provides comfort and orientation to the newly born baby.

The "breast crawl" is a remarkable phenomenon: a baby placed skin-to-skin on the mother's chest immediately after birth will, if left undisturbed and given time (approximately 45 to 60 minutes), crawl up toward the breast and self-attach to the nipple. The baby uses smell, touch, and the visual contrast of the darkened areola to navigate. This self-attachment often results in a better latch than one achieved by positioning the baby manually.

Skin-to-skin is possible after caesarean section, usually in the recovery room, sometimes in the operating theatre itself if the anaesthetist and theatre team permit it. Ask for it. It matters.

Colostrum: The First Milk

For the first 2 to 5 days, your breasts produce colostrum — a thick, golden or yellowish fluid that is quite different from mature breast milk in composition and appearance. Some women worry that "the milk hasn't come in yet" and interpret this as insufficient nutrition for their baby. This is a misunderstanding.

Colostrum is not insufficient. It is specifically designed for the newborn. It is produced in small volumes (5 to 20 mL per feed) precisely because a newborn's stomach capacity is approximately 5 to 7 mL on day 1, expanding to about 22 to 27 mL by day 3. Your colostrum production exactly matches your baby's capacity.

Colostrum is extraordinarily dense in nutrients and immune factors. It is high in proteins and antibodies (particularly secretory IgA, which coats the gut lining and protects against infection), high in fat-soluble vitamins (particularly Vitamin K), and lower in fat and lactose than mature milk — making it easier for the immature neonatal digestive system to handle. It also has a laxative effect, helping to clear meconium from the baby's bowel.

The Milk "Coming In"

At around day 3 to 5, mature milk "comes in" — the transition from colostrum to mature milk that is triggered by the dramatic drop in progesterone following delivery of the placenta. You will know when it happens: your breasts become suddenly and significantly fuller, heavier, and warmer. Some women describe the engorgement as intense — almost painful — in the first 24 to 48 hours.

The single best management for engorgement: feed frequently. Every time your baby feeds, she sends the signal: more milk needed. Your body responds by producing more. This is the supply-demand mechanism that underlies all milk production: supply adjusts to demand, always. Feeding frequently in the early days — 8 to 12 times in 24 hours — establishes your milk supply for weeks and months ahead.

If your baby cannot or will not feed and your breasts are engorged: express by hand or pump to soften the areola, which makes it easier for the baby to latch. Cold compresses between feeds reduce discomfort. Warm compresses or a warm shower immediately before feeding help milk to flow. Cabbage leaves placed inside the bra have genuine anti-inflammatory properties and can reduce severe engorgement — this is not folklore, it has modest clinical evidence.

The Latch: Everything Depends on This

The most common cause of breastfeeding difficulties — cracked nipples, inadequate milk transfer, poor weight gain — is a poor latch. The latch is the way the baby attaches to the breast. A good latch involves the baby taking a large mouthful of breast tissue — not just the nipple — so that the nipple is drawn well back in the baby's mouth, the lower jaw compresses the milk ducts behind the nipple, and milk flows effectively.

Signs of a good latch:

- The baby has a large mouthful of breast — most of the areola, particularly the lower part, is inside the baby's mouth
- The baby's lower lip is flanged outward (like a fish) — not tucked under
- The baby's chin is touching the breast, with nose slightly away from it
- You can hear swallowing — rhythmic, gulping sounds, particularly during the first few minutes when milk is flowing rapidly
- While the initial latch may feel intense for the first few seconds, it should not cause ongoing pain. If it is painful throughout the feed, the latch needs adjustment.

Signs of a poor latch:

- Nipple pain or nipple damage (cracking, bleeding, blistering) after the first few days
- Clicking sounds during feeding (air getting in because the seal is not complete)
- Baby seems constantly hungry despite long feeds
- Baby is not gaining weight adequately

If you suspect a poor latch, ask for a lactation assessment before day 5. A skilled lactation consultant, trained midwife, or breastfeeding support counsellor can observe a feed, identify the specific issue, and give you practical correction — often with immediate improvement.

My NOTE

Breastfeeding can be difficult in the early days. I want to be honest about this because the books that say "breastfeeding should not hurt if done correctly" can make women feel that their pain means they are failing. Sometimes the latch takes time to perfect. Sometimes nipples are genuinely sore for the first week while they adjust. Sometimes a baby has a tongue tie (a tight frenulum that restricts the tongue's range of movement) that interferes with effective feeding. None of this is your fault. Get help early — not at week four when you are exhausted and considering stopping, but at day two when the problem is fresh and solutions are more accessible.

Baby Blues vs Postpartum Depression

There is a spectrum of emotional experience after birth, and understanding where on that spectrum you are — or might be — is one of the most important things in this book.

The Baby Blues

Between day 3 and day 5 after birth — often coinciding with the arrival of milk, which is not a coincidence — approximately 70 to 80% of new mothers experience a wave of emotional vulnerability. Tearfulness, anxiety, irritability, mood swings, the inability to explain why you are crying when your baby is healthy and your husband is trying his best and you have nothing, objectively, to cry about.

This is the baby blues. It is driven by the most dramatic hormonal withdrawal in human physiology — progesterone, which has been at very high levels throughout pregnancy, drops precipitously in the hours after the placenta is delivered. Oestrogen follows. The combined effect is profound emotional vulnerability.

The baby blues resolve spontaneously, typically within 10 to 14 days, without treatment. What helps: rest (as much as a newborn allows), kindness from the people around you, the permission to cry without explanation, and the knowledge that this is normal — not a sign that something is wrong with you or your feelings toward your baby.

Postpartum Depression

Postpartum depression (PPD) is different from the baby blues in several important ways: it does not resolve on its own within two weeks; it is more persistent, deeper, and more disabling; and it requires active treatment.

PPD affects approximately 10 to 15% of women after childbirth. In India, studies suggest the actual prevalence may be higher — possibly 20 to 25% — because of the significant under-reporting that results from cultural pressure to appear happy and grateful after childbirth, stigma around mental health, and limited access to mental health services.

Symptoms of PPD:

- Persistent low mood, sadness, or emptiness lasting more than two weeks
- Loss of interest in things you previously enjoyed, including — and this is hard to say — loss of interest in your baby
- Difficulty bonding with your baby
- Feelings of worthlessness, inadequacy, or guilt — "I am a terrible mother"
- Sleep disturbance beyond what your baby is causing
- Appetite changes — significant loss of appetite, or compulsive eating
- Anxiety that feels uncontrollable — intrusive worries about the baby's health or safety
- Difficulty concentrating or making decisions
- Thoughts of harming yourself or the baby (these require immediate professional support)

PPD is a medical condition. It is not a character flaw. It is not a measure of how much you love your baby. It is not "just hormones" that you should be able to manage by trying harder. It has effective treatments: talking therapies (cognitive behavioural therapy, interpersonal therapy) for mild to moderate cases, and antidepressant medication (sertraline is the first-line choice — it has the most extensive safety data in breastfeeding mothers) for moderate to severe cases. Most women recover fully with appropriate treatment.

" Priya's Fourth Week

"I have a beautiful baby," Priya said, sitting across from me at her four-week check. "My husband loves me. My family is supportive. I have everything I am supposed to want. And I feel nothing. I look at my daughter and I feel — nothing. And then I feel terrified by the nothing. And then I feel like the worst person in the world." She was quiet for a moment. "Nobody told me this could happen." She was not the worst person in the world. She had postpartum depression. We started therapy that week and, six weeks later, sertraline. She sent me a message at three months: "I look at her now and I cannot imagine not feeling this. She is everything. When did this happen?" I wrote back: when you asked for help.

Postpartum Psychosis

Postpartum psychosis is rare — affecting 1 to 2 per 1,000 births — but it is a psychiatric emergency. It typically begins abruptly in the first 1 to 2 weeks after birth. Symptoms include: confusion and disorientation; hallucinations (hearing or seeing things that are not there); delusions (false, fixed beliefs — for example, believing the baby is in danger, or that the mother has special powers, or that family members are impostors); rapid, dramatic mood swings; inability to sleep even when the baby is sleeping; bizarre or very disorganised behaviour.

Postpartum psychosis requires immediate hospital admission and psychiatric treatment. Women with a personal or family history of bipolar disorder are at significantly elevated risk (approximately 25% chance of developing postpartum psychosis). These women should have a specific perinatal mental health plan in place before birth.

If you or your partner notice the symptoms above in the days or weeks after birth: this is an emergency. Call your doctor, go to the emergency department, or call emergency services. The woman experiencing psychosis may not recognise that something is wrong. Act on what you observe.

Your Newborn — What Is Normal

Your baby has arrived from a world of constant warmth, continuous sound, and complete nutritional security into a world of temperature variation, intermittent feeding, and the unmediated bombardment of sensory information. Everything is new. Everything is intense. And almost everything that alarms new parents in the first days and weeks is, in fact, completely normal.

Appearance

Newborns do not always look like the babies in the advertisements. They are beautiful — but with a beauty that takes a moment to appreciate, because they may also be temporarily oddly shaped, blotchy, and covered in substances.

Vernix caseosa: The thick, white, cream cheese-like coating that may cover your baby at birth. It has been protecting her skin throughout the amniotic fluid immersion. It absorbs naturally within hours to days and does not need to be washed off immediately — in fact, leaving it on for a few hours provides ongoing skin protection and moisturising benefit.

Moulding: The elongated, cone-shaped head that results from the skull bones overlapping during passage through the birth canal. It is dramatic to look at and completely resolves within 1 to 3 days as the skull plates return to their normal positions.

Caput succedaneum: Soft swelling of the scalp, usually at the top of the head, caused by fluid accumulation during descent through the birth canal. It crosses the midline of the skull (unlike cephalhaematoma, which is limited to one bone) and typically resolves within a few days.

Milia: Tiny white spots on the nose and cheeks — blocked sebaceous glands. They resolve spontaneously, usually within a few weeks. Do not squeeze them.

Erythema toxicum: An alarming-sounding name for a completely benign rash — blotchy red patches with small yellow or white centres, appearing on the face, trunk, and limbs in the first days. It comes and goes over several days and resolves completely. It is not infectious, not allergic, and requires no treatment.

Mongolian blue spots: Blue-grey, flat birthmarks appearing on the lower back and buttocks, sometimes extending to the limbs. Present in approximately 80 to 90% of South Asian, East Asian, and African newborns. They are caused by melanocytes (pigment cells) in the deep layers of the skin. They fade significantly by age 5 to 10 and are completely benign. Important: document them in the baby's records to prevent any future confusion with bruising.

Neonatal Jaundice

Yellowing of the skin and whites of the eyes (jaundice) appears in approximately 60% of full-term newborns and 80% of premature babies in the first week of life. Most of this is physiological (normal) jaundice, caused by the breakdown of fetal haemoglobin as the baby transitions to adult haemoglobin. The byproduct — bilirubin — accumulates while the newborn liver is still maturing its ability to process it.

Physiological jaundice typically appears on day 2 to 3 (not on day 1 — jaundice appearing within 24 hours of birth is always pathological and warrants urgent investigation), peaks at day 4 to 5, and resolves by day 10 to 14 in full-term babies.

If bilirubin levels rise too high (generally above 350 micromol/L in a term baby, lower thresholds apply in preterm babies), it can cross the blood-brain barrier and cause kernicterus — a form of brain damage causing athetoid cerebral palsy, hearing loss, and intellectual disability. This is preventable with timely treatment.

Treatment: Phototherapy — placing the baby under blue-green lights (430 to 490 nm wavelength) that break down bilirubin in the skin. The baby lies undressed (to maximise skin exposure) with eye protection, for as many hours per day as needed. Most cases of jaundice requiring phototherapy resolve within 1 to 3 days. Exchange transfusion — replacing the baby's blood with donated blood — is reserved for very high or rapidly rising bilirubin levels that do not respond to phototherapy.

✔ WHAT TO DO THIS WEEK

✔ Accept all available help — this is not optional

✔ Sleep when the baby sleeps, even if this goes against all your instincts

✔ Eat regularly — you cannot care for your baby if you are not eating

✔ Do your pelvic floor exercises every day — even small efforts matter

✔ Attend the 6-week postnatal check — for you, not just the baby

✔ Tell someone honestly how you are feeling — do not perform "fine"

✔ If you had a caesarean: follow wound care instructions meticulously

✔ Get help with breastfeeding early if you are struggling — not at week four

✔ Contact your doctor immediately if you develop fever, heavy bleeding, or wound problems

✔ Know the symptoms of postpartum depression and ask for help if needed

7

When Things Are More Complicated

High-Risk Pregnancy and Warning Signs

The vast majority of pregnancies are uncomplicated. I want you to begin this chapter with that fact clearly in mind: most women go through pregnancy without a significant medical complication, give birth to a healthy baby, and recover without lasting consequences. That is the most likely story for you.

But some pregnancies are more complex. And if yours is one of them — or if you simply want to understand the conditions your doctor screens for at every appointment — this chapter will give you the honest, clear information you deserve.

Knowledge is not frightening. The fear comes from uncertainty — from not understanding what a diagnosis means, what the treatment involves, or what the realistic outcomes are. Clear information replaces uncertainty with understanding. And understanding, even of difficult things, is always better than ignorance.

Pre-Eclampsia

Pre-eclampsia is a condition unique to pregnancy — it cannot occur outside of it. It is defined by the development of high blood pressure (hypertension) after 20 weeks of pregnancy, accompanied by signs of organ involvement — most commonly protein in the urine (proteinuria) indicating kidney involvement, but also elevation of liver enzymes, reduction in platelet count, neurological symptoms, or evidence of fetal compromise.

It affects approximately 5 to 8% of pregnancies globally — perhaps slightly higher in India, where baseline rates of hypertension and metabolic syndrome are elevated in the reproductive-age population. It is the leading cause of maternal mortality and morbidity in high-income countries, and a major contributor in India.

Why Does Pre-Eclampsia Happen?

Pre-eclampsia begins with abnormal implantation of the placenta. In a normal pregnancy, the trophoblast cells of the early placenta invade deeply into the spiral arteries of the uterus, widening them into low-resistance, high-flow vessels that can accommodate the enormous increase in blood flow needed to sustain fetal growth. In pre-eclampsia, this invasion is incomplete — the spiral arteries remain narrow, high-resistance vessels.

The result is a placenta under chronic ischaemic (low oxygen) stress. This stressed placenta releases a range of factors — including sFlt-1 (an anti-angiogenic protein) and inflammatory cytokines — into the maternal circulation. These circulating factors damage the endothelial cells (lining cells) of blood vessels throughout the body, causing widespread vascular dysfunction: high blood pressure, leaky capillaries (causing protein to spill into urine and fluid to leak into tissues), platelet activation, and impaired function of the liver, kidneys, and brain.

This explains why the cure for pre-eclampsia is delivery of the placenta — the source of the problem. After the placenta is delivered, blood pressure typically normalises within days to weeks.

Types and Severity

Pre-eclampsia without severe features (previously called "mild" pre-eclampsia) is characterised by blood pressure of 140/90 mmHg or higher on two readings at least 4 hours apart, with proteinuria (protein/creatinine ratio above 30 mg/mmol, or 300 mg/24 hours), without the features of severe disease. It can be managed with close monitoring and may not require immediate delivery if remote from term.

Pre-eclampsia with severe features requires more urgent management and includes: blood pressure of 160/110 mmHg or higher; platelets below 100 x 10^9/L; elevated liver enzymes with right upper quadrant pain; serum creatinine above 97 micromol/L; pulmonary oedema; new-onset severe headache; visual disturbances.

HELLP syndrome — Haemolysis (destruction of red blood cells), Elevated Liver enzymes, and Low Platelets — is a severe variant of pre-eclampsia that requires urgent delivery regardless of gestational age.

Eclampsia is pre-eclampsia complicated by grand mal seizures. It is a medical emergency. Magnesium sulphate, the treatment of choice, both treats the seizures and prevents their recurrence more effectively than anticonvulsants.

Can Pre-Eclampsia Be Prevented?

For women identified as high risk (previous pre-eclampsia, chronic hypertension, renal disease, diabetes, multiple pregnancy, or first-trimester combined screening showing elevated sFlt-1/PlGF ratio), low-dose aspirin 150 mg daily, started before 16 weeks of pregnancy, reduces the risk of preterm pre-eclampsia by approximately 60 to 80% (ASPRE trial, 2017). This is one of the most significant advances in preventive obstetrics of the past decade.

Calcium supplementation (1.5 to 2 grams daily) in women with low dietary calcium intake — which includes the majority of Indian women — also reduces the risk of pre-eclampsia by approximately 50% (WHO recommendation, Cochrane meta-analysis). This is inexpensive, safe, and widely ignored. Ask your doctor about it.

Symptoms of Pre-Eclampsia — See Your Doctor Today

These symptoms in the second or third trimester require same-day assessment:

- A severe headache that does not respond to paracetamol — persistent, frontal or generalised
- Visual disturbances: blurring, flashing lights, spots, temporary loss of vision
- Pain or tenderness in the upper right abdomen or under the ribs (liver involvement)

• Sudden, significant swelling of the face, hands, or feet — beyond normal pregnancy oedema

• Feeling generally very unwell in a way you cannot explain

• Nausea and vomiting in the third trimester (not early pregnancy nausea)

None of these alone confirms pre-eclampsia. All of them deserve the same-day attention.

Miscarriage

Miscarriage is the loss of a pregnancy before 24 weeks. It is the most common complication of pregnancy, affecting approximately 15 to 20% of all confirmed pregnancies. The true rate is higher — many very early losses occur before a missed period, unrecognised as pregnancies. Studies using daily sensitive blood tests estimate that 30 to 40% of all fertilised eggs are lost before becoming clinical pregnancies.

The vast majority of miscarriages — approximately 75% — occur in the first trimester. After a heartbeat has been confirmed on scan at 8 to 10 weeks, the ongoing risk of miscarriage drops to approximately 2 to 5%.

Why Miscarriage Happens

The most important thing I can tell you about miscarriage — and I say this having sat with hundreds of women in the aftermath of one — is what did not cause it.

It was not caused by exercise. It was not caused by working too hard, or not resting enough, or carrying something heavy. It was not caused by stress, or an argument, or a frightening event. It was not caused by the food you ate, or the food you did not eat. It was not caused by sex. It was not caused by anything you did or failed to do.

Approximately 60 to 70% of first-trimester miscarriages are caused by chromosomal abnormalities in the embryo — random errors in the division of chromosomes at or around fertilisation.

The embryo, carrying these errors, develops abnormally. The pregnancy ends. This is the body's quality-control system working — imperfect, devastating, but not the result of any action of the mother.

The remainder of early miscarriages are caused by a range of factors: uterine abnormalities (fibroids, a septum), thrombophilia (clotting disorders), immunological conditions (antiphospholipid syndrome), poorly controlled thyroid disease, severe diabetes, or — in older women — the higher rate of chromosomal abnormality in eggs.

What Happens During a Miscarriage

A miscarriage may be identified in several ways: by vaginal bleeding (which may be light spotting or heavy flow with clots), by cramping lower abdominal pain, by the disappearance of pregnancy symptoms, or — in a missed or silent miscarriage — entirely on ultrasound scan with no symptoms at all.

A missed miscarriage is when the embryo has stopped developing but the uterus has not yet expelled the pregnancy — the pregnancy sac is present, but there is no fetal heartbeat. This can be particularly difficult psychologically because there are no symptoms to prepare you — you may feel entirely pregnant until the moment the scan reveals otherwise.

Management options for a confirmed miscarriage:

Expectant management: Waiting for the miscarriage to complete naturally. The majority of first-trimester miscarriages will complete within two weeks if managed expectantly. This is appropriate for stable women who prefer to avoid medical intervention and are counselled about the signs of incomplete miscarriage (prolonged heavy bleeding, fever).

Medical management: Misoprostol tablets — given vaginally, sublingually, or orally — stimulate uterine contractions to expel the pregnancy. Effective in approximately 80% of cases within 1 to 2 days. Side effects include cramping, nausea, and diarrhoea.

Surgical management: Manual vacuum aspiration (MVA) or surgical evacuation of the uterus under local or general anaesthesia. Effective, rapid, and appropriate when the woman prefers it, when medical management has failed, or when there are clinical concerns (very heavy bleeding, suspected infection).

✍ My NOTE

Recurrent miscarriage — three or more consecutive pregnancy losses — affects approximately 1 to 2% of couples trying to conceive. I want to address this specifically because the grief of recurrent loss is profound and is often inadequately supported. Investigation for recurrent miscarriage includes: uterine imaging (to exclude structural abnormalities), karyotyping of both partners (to identify chromosomal translocations), antiphospholipid antibody testing, thrombophilia screen, and thyroid function. In approximately 50% of couples, no cause is found — which is frustrating, but does not mean the next pregnancy will be lost. With appropriate support, approximately 70% of women with unexplained recurrent miscarriage achieve a successful ongoing pregnancy.

Preterm Labour and Birth

Preterm birth — delivery before 37 completed weeks of gestation — affects approximately 10% of pregnancies globally and is the leading cause of neonatal mortality (death in the first 28 days of life) and a major cause of long-term neurodevelopmental disability.

Preterm birth is divided into:

- Extremely preterm: before 28 weeks — highest mortality and morbidity
- Very preterm: 28 to 31+6 weeks — significant neonatal intensive care required
- Moderate to late preterm: 32 to 36+6 weeks — most common, generally good outcomes with appropriate care

Risk factors include: previous preterm birth (the single strongest risk factor), multiple pregnancy, uterine abnormalities, cervical shortening, bacterial vaginosis, urinary tract infection, maternal stress, smoking, very low or very high BMI, and certain racial and socioeconomic factors.

Cervical Length Screening

Women at high risk of preterm birth (particularly those with a previous preterm birth) are offered cervical length measurement by transvaginal ultrasound at 18 to 24 weeks. A short cervix — below 25 mm — is associated with a significantly elevated risk of preterm birth and is the strongest ultrasound predictor of preterm labour.

Women with a short cervix (less than 25 mm) between 18 and 24 weeks who are not currently pregnant with twins are offered vaginal progesterone — 200 mg pessary nightly, inserted vaginally. This is one of the most evidence-based interventions in modern obstetrics: vaginal progesterone in women with a short cervix reduces the rate of preterm birth before 33 weeks by approximately 45% (Fonseca et al., New England Journal of Medicine, 2007).

Cervical cerclage — a surgical stitch placed around the cervix to reinforce it — is considered in women with a very short cervix (less than 15 mm) or a history of recurrent mid-trimester pregnancy loss or previous preterm birth attributed to cervical insufficiency.

If Preterm Labour Begins

If regular contractions or ruptured membranes occur before 34 weeks: go to hospital immediately. Do not wait and see. The following interventions significantly improve neonatal outcomes when given before 34 weeks:

Antenatal corticosteroids (betamethasone 12 mg IM, two doses 24 hours apart, or dexamethasone 6 mg IM, four doses 12 hours apart): Dramatically accelerate fetal lung maturation, reducing the risk of respiratory distress syndrome (RDS) by 40%, intraventricular haemorrhage (bleeding in the brain) by 50%, and neonatal death by 30%. This is one of the most effective and cost-effective interventions in all of medicine. It requires 24 to 48 hours to take full effect — hence the urgency of arriving at hospital promptly.

Tocolysis: Medications (nifedipine, atosiban, indomethacin) used to temporarily halt or slow uterine contractions, buying time for the corticosteroids to take effect and for transfer to a hospital with a neonatal unit.

Magnesium sulphate: Given to women threatening preterm birth before 32 weeks, not to stop labour, but for neuroprotection of the fetal brain — it reduces the risk of cerebral palsy in very preterm survivors by approximately 30%.

Placenta Praevia and Accreta

Placenta praevia occurs when the placenta is located in the lower segment of the uterus, either partially or completely covering the internal cervical os (the opening of the cervix). It affects approximately 0.3 to 0.5% of pregnancies at term — a low absolute rate, but a clinically important condition because it causes antepartum haemorrhage and precludes vaginal delivery.

Most low-lying placentas identified at the 20-week scan migrate upward as the uterus grows — because the upper segment of the uterus expands differentially more than the lower segment. By 32 to 36 weeks, only a minority of women with a low-lying placenta at 20 weeks still have praevia. For this reason, a follow-up scan at 32 to 34 weeks is recommended for all women in whom the placenta was noted to be low at the anomaly scan.

Major placenta praevia (covering the os) at term requires planned caesarean section — usually at 36 to 37 weeks, before spontaneous labour begins. Vaginal delivery with praevia risks catastrophic haemorrhage as the lower segment effaces and dilates. Any vaginal bleeding in a woman with known praevia must be treated as a potential emergency — go to hospital immediately, do not drive yourself.

Placenta accreta spectrum describes the abnormal invasion of placental trophoblast into the myometrium (uterine muscle) and beyond. It ranges from accreta (superficial myometrial invasion), to increta (invasion through the myometrium), to percreta (through the uterine wall, potentially into adjacent organs including the bladder and bowel). It is a serious condition, associated with massive haemorrhage at delivery, and its incidence is rising — primarily as a consequence of rising caesarean section rates. Each previous caesarean scar creates a defect through which placental tissue can invade in subsequent pregnancies.

Management requires a multidisciplinary team: MFM specialist, experienced obstetric surgeon, interventional radiologist, urologist, and blood bank. Delivery in a tertiary centre with planned preoperative preparation is associated with significantly lower maternal morbidity and mortality.

Anaemia in Pregnancy

Iron-deficiency anaemia in pregnancy is India's most common and most consequential pregnancy complication. It affects more than 50% of pregnant Indian women according to NFHS-5 (2019-21) — a figure that has barely moved in decades despite government supplementation programmes.

The consequences of anaemia in pregnancy are severe and underappreciated. Maternal consequences: increased risk of postpartum haemorrhage (because an anaemic woman starts with reduced haemoglobin reserves and therefore tolerates even normal blood loss less well), increased susceptibility to infection, increased risk of cardiac failure in severe cases, and reduced tolerance of the physiological demands of labour. Neonatal consequences: preterm birth, low birth weight, and iron-deficiency anaemia in the infant (fetal iron stores are established in the third trimester from maternal iron, so maternal deficiency directly causes neonatal deficiency).

THE SCIENCE BEHIND IT

The Iron Absorption Problem in India

Why is iron deficiency so prevalent in India despite iron being present in the diet? The answer lies in the form of iron available and the factors that affect its absorption.

There are two forms of dietary iron:

Haem iron: Found in meat, poultry, and fish. Absorbed at 15 to 35% regardless of body iron status or dietary factors. The most bioavailable form.

Non-haem iron: Found in all plant foods — legumes, leafy vegetables, grains, nuts. Absorbed at only 2 to 5% under baseline conditions. Highly susceptible to inhibitors and enhancers.

For the predominantly vegetarian Indian diet, essentially all dietary iron is non-haem. Its absorption is profoundly inhibited by:

- Phytates: Present in whole grains, legumes, and cereals — the staples of the Indian diet
- Polyphenols: Present in tea and coffee — consumed with or after most Indian meals

• Calcium: Competes with iron for absorption — a problem when iron tablets are taken with milk

• Concurrent infections: Inflammation suppresses iron absorption and utilisation

Non-haem iron absorption is powerfully enhanced by Vitamin C (ascorbic acid), which reduces ferric iron to the more bioavailable ferrous form. The combination of a squeeze of lemon on dahl or a glass of amla juice with an iron tablet can increase absorption from 2% to 15-20% — a 7 to 10 fold improvement.

Amla (Indian gooseberry, Phyllanthus emblica) contains 600 to 700 mg of Vitamin C per 100g — the highest concentration of any commonly available food in India, and one of the highest of any food in the world. Even a small amla (about 10g) provides 60-70 mg of Vitamin C. Eating amla with iron-rich meals is not folk wisdom — it is biochemistry.

Mental Health Conditions in Pregnancy

Psychiatric illness — depression, anxiety, PTSD, bipolar disorder, schizophrenia — does not spare pregnant women. In fact, pregnancy and the postpartum period represent a time of elevated vulnerability to several mental health conditions, due to the combination of hormonal changes, physical demands, sleep disruption, identity transition, and social pressures.

Antenatal depression affects approximately 10 to 12% of pregnant women — a prevalence similar to postnatal depression but far less recognised and discussed. Antenatal anxiety, including panic disorder, generalised anxiety disorder, and obsessive-compulsive presentations, may be even more common. Tokophobia — a severe, debilitating fear of childbirth — affects approximately 6 to 10% of women and can range from distressing to functionally incapacitating.

Untreated mental health conditions in pregnancy have real consequences: for the mother's wellbeing, for her ability to engage with antenatal care, for the couple's relationship, and — through the effects of stress hormones and poor self-care — for the fetus. The risk of untreated depression is not less than the risk of treatment. They must be weighed honestly.

The Edinburgh Postnatal Depression Scale (EPDS) is a validated 10-question tool used to screen for depression in pregnancy and the postpartum period. Your doctor should administer it at the booking visit and again at 28 weeks. If you are struggling emotionally at any point in pregnancy, please say so. The question "how are you feeling emotionally?" at antenatal appointments is not a pleasantry — it is a clinical assessment.

Treatment: Mild to moderate antenatal depression and anxiety are treated with structured psychological therapy — cognitive behavioural therapy (CBT) is the most evidence-based approach, and brief CBT is effective and can be delivered by trained counsellors in Indian settings. Moderate to severe conditions, or those unresponsive to therapy alone, may require antidepressant medication. Sertraline is the preferred first-line antidepressant in pregnancy and lactation — it has the most extensive safety data, the lowest measured levels in breast milk, and no established association with significant congenital malformation at standard doses.

8

Eating Well, the Indian Way

Nutrition Throughout Your Pregnancy

"You are eating for two now." Your mother, your mother-in-law, your neighbour, the fruit vendor who has known you since you were a child — they will all say some version of this. And they mean well. But the advice, as given, is not quite right.

You are not eating twice as much. You are eating for the growth of a human nervous system, a human skeleton, a human immune system, and a human heart — none of which can be built from extra chapatis alone. What you need is not more food in general, but the right food, consistently, across all three trimesters.

The good news — and I mean this genuinely — is that traditional Indian home cooking, at its best, is extraordinarily well-designed for pregnancy. Dahl and rice together form a complete protein. Turmeric is one of the most extensively studied anti-inflammatory substances in nutritional science. Methi seeds and leaves are rich in iron, calcium, and fibre. Sesame (til) is among the richest plant sources of calcium on the planet. Amla is the richest known source of Vitamin C. Our traditional thali, if composed thoughtfully, contains almost everything a pregnant woman needs.

The problem is not traditional food. The problem is the replacement of traditional food with processed, refined, and convenience-oriented alternatives — white bread, packaged biscuits, maida-heavy snacks, cold drinks — that are calorie-dense and nutritionally empty. Pregnancy is the best possible reason to return to the kitchen.

How Much Extra Do You Actually Need?

The caloric requirement of pregnancy is often dramatically overstated. The actual additional caloric need:

- First trimester: Approximately 0 extra calories per day. Yes, zero. Your body becomes more efficient at extracting nutrients from food in early pregnancy, and the embryo is too small to have significant caloric needs. If you are eating normally — or even less, because of nausea — your baby is not going hungry.

- Second trimester: Approximately 340 extra calories per day. This is less than a small additional meal — roughly equivalent to a bowl of dahl and two rotis, or a cup of dahi with fruit and a handful of nuts.
- Third trimester: Approximately 450 extra calories per day. Still a modest increase.

The obsession with eating "for two" is one of the reasons gestational diabetes, excessive gestational weight gain, and macrosomia (very large babies) are becoming more common. Quality, not quantity, is the prescription.

Protein: The Building Block You Cannot Skip

Protein requirements increase significantly in pregnancy: from approximately 46 to 50 grams per day before pregnancy to 71 to 80 grams per day during pregnancy (ICMR-NIN 2020 recommendations for Indian women). Protein is essential for fetal growth, placental development, expansion of maternal blood volume, and the growth of uterine and breast tissue.

Excellent protein sources for Indian women, with rough amounts per serving:

- Dahl (cooked, 1 cup / 200g): 9 grams protein. Different dals have slightly different profiles — masoor (red lentil), moong (green/yellow lentil), chana (chickpea), and urad (black lentil) are all excellent. Eat dahl at least twice daily.
- Paneer (100g): 18 grams protein. One of the most protein-dense plant-based foods available in India. Homemade paneer from full-fat cow's milk is ideal.
- Dahi / curd (1 cup / 150g): 8 grams protein. Also excellent for calcium and probiotics.
- Eggs (1 whole egg): 6 grams protein. The most bioavailable protein source available — the reference standard against which all other proteins are measured. Two eggs daily is a

nutritionally excellent contribution to pregnancy protein needs.

- Chicken (100g cooked): 27 grams protein. Chicken, particularly lean chicken breast, is an outstanding pregnancy food — high protein, high iron, low saturated fat.
- Fish (100g): 20 to 25 grams protein, plus omega-3 fatty acids. Choose low-mercury fish: rohu, katla, pomfret, sardines, mackerel (bangda). Avoid high-mercury fish: swordfish, shark, king mackerel, tilefish.
- Rajma / kidney beans (1 cup cooked, 170g): 15 grams protein. Also excellent for iron and fibre.
- Soya (100g tofu, or 1/2 cup cooked soya beans): 10 to 17 grams protein. Safe in normal dietary amounts during pregnancy.
- Milk (1 glass / 250 mL): 8 grams protein plus calcium. Always boil fresh milk before drinking.

Iron: The Imperative

Iron requirements in pregnancy nearly double: from approximately 18 mg per day before pregnancy to 27 mg per day during pregnancy. In the third trimester, when fetal iron stores are being established, demand peaks. Indian women begin pregnancy with already depleted iron stores in the majority of cases — the gap between requirement and intake is enormous.

Iron-rich foods to eat daily:

- Dark green leafy vegetables: Palak (spinach), methi (fenugreek), moringa/drumstick leaves (sahjan patti), amaranth (rajgira/chauli), bathua. Moringa leaves deserve special mention: they contain 28 mg of iron per 100g of dry powder — extraordinary for a plant food. A teaspoon of moringa powder added to dahl or chapati dough daily is a meaningful contribution.
- Legumes: All lentils and beans. Masoor dahl has the highest iron content among common dals.

- Jaggery (gud): 11 mg iron per 100g — far higher than refined sugar (which has essentially none). Substituting jaggery for sugar in tea, sweets, and cooking is a simple, culturally consistent way to increase iron intake.
- Ragi (finger millet): 3.9 mg iron per 100g. One of the most nutritionally impressive grains available in India — high in iron, high in calcium, high in fibre, low glycaemic index. Ragi rotis, ragi dosas, ragi porridge with jaggery — all are excellent pregnancy foods.
- Til (sesame seeds): 14.5 mg iron per 100g. A tablespoon of sesame seeds added to doughs, chutneys, or sprinkled over vegetables makes a genuine nutritional difference.
- Liver: Goat liver (kaleji) is the single richest dietary source of iron — 6 to 8 mg per 100g, in the highly bioavailable haem form. Limit to once a week because of high Vitamin A content (excess retinol in the first trimester is teratogenic at very high intakes from supplements, though dietary sources are generally safe at normal consumption).

Always eat iron-rich plant foods with Vitamin C: a squeeze of lemon, a small amla, a piece of guava, half a raw tomato. The conversion of non-haem iron from ferric to ferrous form — facilitated by Vitamin C — is the most significant single factor determining whether the iron in your food is actually absorbed.

Always take iron supplements away from tea, coffee, and calcium: all of these significantly inhibit iron absorption. Take your IFA (iron-folic acid) tablet either on an empty stomach (if your stomach tolerates it) or with a glass of amla juice — not with breakfast chai.

Calcium: Beyond Just Milk

Calcium requirements increase in pregnancy: 1,000 to 1,300 mg daily. Your baby needs approximately 30 grams of calcium across the pregnancy for bone and tooth development. If your diet does not provide it, she will take it from your bones — increasing your long-term risk of osteoporosis.

Many Indian women do not drink enough milk to meet calcium requirements — due to lactose intolerance, taste, cost, or habit. Excellent alternative calcium sources:

- Ragi (finger millet): 344 mg calcium per 100g — the richest plant source of calcium readily available in India. More calcium than milk, gram for gram. One ragi roti (approximately 30g dry weight) provides over 100 mg calcium. A daily ragi preparation is one of the most impactful single dietary changes an Indian pregnant woman can make.
- Til (sesame seeds): 975 mg calcium per 100g. Extraordinary. Even a tablespoon (15g) provides nearly 150 mg — 15% of the daily requirement. Make til ladoos, add sesame to chutneys, sprinkle on salads.
- Moringa (drumstick leaves): 440 mg calcium per 100g dry weight. Add to dahl, parathas, or eggs.
- Amaranth leaves (rajgira / chauli): 397 mg calcium per 100g. Widely available, inexpensive, underused.
- Paneer: 208 mg per 100g. One good serving of paneer sabzi daily provides meaningful calcium.
- Full-fat dahi (curd): 150 to 200 mg per 100g. A bowl of dahi after lunch is calcium, protein, and probiotics in a single preparation.
- Dried figs (anjeer): 162 mg calcium per 100g. A handful of soaked figs as a snack is a simple calcium supplement.

WHO recommends 1.5 to 2 grams of calcium supplementation daily in populations with low dietary calcium intake — which includes the majority of India. Ask your doctor about calcium supplementation from the second trimester onwards.

Vitamin D: India's Paradox

India receives more sunlight than almost any country on earth. And yet Vitamin D deficiency affects an estimated 70 to 90% of Indian pregnant women. This is not a contradiction — it is the result of a specific constellation of factors that are largely unique to India:

Sun exposure in India is high, but skin exposure is limited. Most Indian women cover their arms and legs for cultural or practical reasons. When sunscreen is used, it blocks Vitamin D synthesis. Urban air pollution reduces the UV-B radiation reaching the skin. Many women spend the majority of their daylight hours indoors.

The diet contains almost no Vitamin D. Vitamin D3 is found in significant amounts in only a handful of foods: oily fish (mackerel, sardines, salmon), egg yolks, and fortified products (some milks, some cereals). For a predominantly vegetarian Indian diet, dietary Vitamin D is essentially absent.

Darker skin requires more sun exposure to produce the same amount of Vitamin D as lighter skin — because melanin (the pigment responsible for darker skin colour) competes with 7-dehydrocholesterol (the precursor to Vitamin D) for UV-B photons.

The consequences of Vitamin D deficiency in pregnancy are serious: increased risk of pre-eclampsia, gestational diabetes, preterm birth, low birth weight, and neonatal rickets (soft, weak bones in the newborn). The baby's entire Vitamin D store at birth comes from the mother.

Supplementation: FOGSI and the Indian Academy of Pediatrics recommend supplementing all pregnant Indian women with 1,000 to 2,000 IU of Vitamin D3 daily throughout pregnancy. This is safe at these doses and dramatically improves outcomes in deficient populations.

Folate: Beyond Just the First Trimester

Folic acid supplementation in the pre-conception period and first trimester is essential for neural tube closure, as discussed extensively in Chapter 1. But folate requirements remain elevated throughout pregnancy — the developing fetal nervous system continues to need folate for cell division and DNA synthesis.

400 mcg supplemental folic acid daily is the standard recommendation from before conception through 12 weeks. After 12 weeks, the WHO and FOGSI recommend continuing folic acid (usually as part of an IFA supplement — iron-folic acid) throughout pregnancy.

Dietary folate sources for Indian women: green leafy vegetables (methi, palak, moringa leaves — all excellent), legumes (particularly masoor dahl and rajma), citrus fruits, amla, papaya (ripe), and whole grains. Cooking destroys folate; lightly cooked or raw vegetables have higher folate content than thoroughly boiled ones.

Foods to Avoid in Pregnancy

The list of things pregnant women are told to avoid is often far longer than necessary, generating anxiety without benefit. Here is what the evidence actually supports:

- Alcohol: None. No safe amount has been established. Fetal alcohol spectrum disorder represents a continuum of neurodevelopmental damage; the lower end of this spectrum — subtle cognitive and behavioural effects — may occur at exposures below those that cause obvious physical features. Abstain completely.
- Raw or undercooked meat and eggs: Risk of toxoplasma (from undercooked meat) and salmonella (from raw eggs). Ensure all meat and eggs are thoroughly cooked. Runny eggs (half-boiled, sunny side up) are a mild risk — avoid them if you have any doubts about egg freshness.
- Raw papaya (kachchi papita): Contains papain and prostaglandins that may stimulate uterine contractions. Avoid raw, green, unripe papaya throughout pregnancy. Ripe, soft orange papaya in normal dietary amounts is safe and nutritious — rich in Vitamin C, Vitamin A, and folate.

- High-mercury fish: Swordfish, shark, king mackerel, tilefish — avoid. These bioaccumulate mercury, a neurotoxin, in their fat. Low-mercury Indian fish (rohu, katla, pomfret, bangda, sardines) are excellent pregnancy foods and should be eaten regularly.
- Excess caffeine: Above 200 mg per day is associated with increased miscarriage risk. One strong cup of filter coffee: approximately 200 mg. Standard chai: 25 to 50 mg per cup. Two to three cups of tea daily is fine; multiple strong coffees are not.
- Unpasteurised milk (kacha doodh): Risk of listeria, brucellosis, and other bacterial infections. Always boil fresh milk before use.
- Pre-cut fruit and street food: The infection risk from contamination is real, particularly listeria (which can cause fetal infection, miscarriage, and stillbirth) and E. coli. If buying cut fruit from vendors, choose freshly cut fruit where you can see it being cut. Be cautious about water sources.
- Excess Vitamin A from animal sources (retinol): Very high doses of preformed Vitamin A (retinol) — typically only achieved through high-dose supplements or liver consumed in large quantities daily — are teratogenic in the first trimester. Normal dietary liver (once a week) and normal dietary beta-carotene (from vegetables and fruits) are safe. Do not take high-dose retinol supplements.

What is safe that rumour says is not: spicy food (does not harm the baby; may worsen your heartburn), pineapple in normal amounts (bromelain in food quantities is safe; bromelain supplements in very high doses are different), mangoes, papaya (ripe), tomatoes, turmeric in cooking quantities — virtually all Indian spices are safe in normal culinary quantities.

" Sunita's Mango Anxiety

"My mother-in-law told me I cannot eat mangoes," Sunita said at her 18-week appointment. "She says they are heating foods and will cause miscarriage." She looked genuinely distressed — she is from Ratnagiri and mangoes are practically her religion. I told her: mangoes are among the most nutritious fruits available in India. They are rich in Vitamin C, Vitamin A (beta-carotene form), folate, and potassium. They are safe in pregnancy. The concept of "heating" and "cooling" foods is a cultural framework, not a medical one, and has no evidence base in relation to miscarriage or pregnancy complications. She asked if she could tell her mother-in-law I said so. I told her: yes, with pleasure.

9

Medicines, Safety, and a Final Word

What Is Safe, What Is Not, and the Journey Ahead

Medicines in pregnancy generate an enormous amount of anxiety — and for good reason. The thalidomide tragedy of the 1950s and 1960s, in which a sedative drug caused severe limb defects in thousands of children born to mothers who had taken it in early pregnancy, established in the public consciousness a fear of any medication during pregnancy that persists to this day.

That fear, however, has a shadow side: it leads women to suffer unnecessarily (refusing to take safe medication for fever, pain, or nausea because "I don't want to take anything in pregnancy"), and occasionally to stop prescribed medication that is genuinely necessary — sometimes with serious consequences.

The reality is more nuanced than "all medication is dangerous in pregnancy." Many medications are entirely safe. Many are safe at specific gestational ages. Some are genuinely dangerous. And a small number are absolutely contraindicated. Understanding the difference is important.

How Medications Affect Pregnancy

Whether a medication affects the fetus depends on several factors:

Does it cross the placenta? Most small molecules can cross the placenta to some extent. Larger molecules (like most proteins and some injectable drugs) cross poorly or not at all. The degree of crossing is proportional to the concentration in maternal blood and the lipid solubility of the drug.

At what gestational age is it taken? The embryonic period (weeks 3 to 8) is the most sensitive window — when major structural malformations can occur. After 12 weeks, the risk of structural birth defects from most medications drops significantly, though functional effects on developing organs (brain, kidneys, reproductive system) remain possible.

What dose and for how long? Brief exposure to a low dose of most medications is typically far less concerning than prolonged high-dose exposure.

Medicines That Are Safe in Pregnancy

Paracetamol

Paracetamol (acetaminophen) is the safest analgesic and antipyretic available in pregnancy. It can be taken in all three trimesters at standard doses (500 mg to 1 g, up to four times daily) for short-term treatment of fever, headache, and pain. It should be used at the lowest effective dose for the shortest duration necessary. Recent epidemiological studies have raised questions about prolonged paracetamol use and neurodevelopmental outcomes — but these are observational studies with many confounders, and current guidance from FOGSI, RCOG, and ACOG continues to endorse short-term use as safe.

Fever itself — above 38°C — is harmful to the developing fetus, particularly in the first trimester. Treating fever promptly with paracetamol is important. Do not leave significant fever untreated because of concerns about paracetamol.

Antacids

Calcium carbonate antacids (Gelusil, Digene, Eno) are safe throughout pregnancy. Magnesium trisilicate should be avoided in high doses. Proton pump inhibitors (omeprazole, pantoprazole) are used when antacids are insufficient and are considered safe for short courses. Ranitidine (H2 blocker) was widely used in pregnancy until concerns about NDMA contamination; famotidine is the preferred H2 blocker currently.

Iron and Vitamins

All standard pregnancy vitamins and supplements — folic acid, iron, calcium, Vitamin D, Vitamin B12 — are safe throughout pregnancy at recommended doses. High-dose Vitamin A (retinol form, above 10,000 IU daily from supplements) should be avoided in the first trimester due to teratogenicity at very high doses. Beta-carotene (plant-source Vitamin A) is safe at any dose.

Antibiotics

Several antibiotics are safe throughout pregnancy:

- Amoxicillin, amoxicillin-clavulanate (Augmentin): Safe in all trimesters. First-line treatment for urinary tract infections and respiratory infections.
- Cephalosporins (cefalexin, cefuroxime, ceftriaxone): Safe in all trimesters.
- Clindamycin: Safe. Used for bacterial vaginosis and skin infections.
- Azithromycin: Generally considered safe, with more caution in the first trimester where data is more limited.
- Nitrofurantoin: Safe in the first and second trimester for urinary tract infections; avoid near term (after 36 weeks) due to risk of neonatal haemolytic anaemia.

Antibiotics to avoid in pregnancy:

- Tetracyclines (doxycycline): Permanently stain and damage developing teeth and bones. Contraindicated from the second trimester onwards.
- Fluoroquinolones (ciprofloxacin, levofloxacin): Associated with cartilage damage in animal studies; avoided in pregnancy unless no safe alternative exists.
- Trimethoprim: Folate antagonist — avoid in the first trimester.
- Sulfonamides (trimethoprim-sulfamethoxazole): Avoid in the first trimester (folate antagonism) and at term (neonatal jaundice).

Medicines That Are Dangerous in Pregnancy

NSAIDs After 20 Weeks

Non-steroidal anti-inflammatory drugs — ibuprofen, diclofenac, naproxen, aspirin in anti-inflammatory doses — are safe in the first and early second trimester for short-term use. However, from 20 weeks onwards, they must be avoided. After 20 weeks, NSAIDs can cause premature closure of the ductus arteriosus (a critical blood vessel in the fetal circulation whose closure at birth is normally triggered by the newborn's first breaths) and oligohydramnios (reduction in amniotic fluid from decreased fetal urine output — because NSAIDs impair fetal kidney function). Both are serious, potentially irreversible conditions. Low-dose aspirin (75 to 150 mg for pre-eclampsia prevention) is a specific exception with established safety.

ACE Inhibitors and ARBs

ACE inhibitors (enalapril, lisinopril, ramipril) and angiotensin receptor blockers (losartan, valsartan, telmisartan) — commonly used for hypertension and kidney disease — are teratogenic in the second and third trimesters. They cause fetal renal tubular dysplasia, oligohydramnios, skull ossification defects, and fetal death. Any woman on these medications who is pregnant or planning pregnancy must switch to a pregnancy-safe antihypertensive (labetalol, nifedipine, methyldopa, hydralazine) as soon as possible.

Valproate

Sodium valproate (used for epilepsy and bipolar disorder) is associated with a 6 to 10% risk of major congenital malformations (neural tube defects, cardiac defects, cleft palate, hypospadias) and a 30 to 40% risk of neurodevelopmental problems in the child (autism, intellectual disability, ADHD, language delays). It is the most teratogenic commonly prescribed medication in use in India. Every woman of reproductive age taking valproate should have a documented, informed discussion with her prescribing doctor about alternatives — alternatives exist for most indications. If valproate is genuinely the only effective treatment, the woman must use highly effective contraception and, if pregnancy is desired, make the decision in consultation with a neurologist or psychiatrist and a maternal-fetal medicine specialist.

Warfarin

Warfarin (used for anticoagulation in women with mechanical heart valves, thrombophilia, or previous clotting events) crosses the placenta and causes warfarin embryopathy in the first trimester (nasal hypoplasia, limb abnormalities, eye abnormalities). It also causes fetal haemorrhage throughout pregnancy due to its anticoagulant effect on the fetus. Management: switch to low-molecular-weight heparin (LMWH, which does not cross the placenta) in the first trimester and at term. Women with mechanical heart valves — who have very high thrombotic risk — have a complex risk-benefit calculation that requires individual specialist input.

Isotretinoin

Isotretinoin (Roaccutane, Acutret) — used for severe acne — is one of the most potently teratogenic substances known. A single course of treatment at therapeutic doses during the first trimester carries a 25 to 35% risk of major congenital malformations (craniofacial, cardiac, thymic, central nervous system) and approximately 25% risk of spontaneous miscarriage. Pregnancy must be absolutely excluded before starting treatment, and two forms of contraception must be used throughout. Do not attempt conception for at least one month after the last dose.

Vaccinations in Pregnancy

Vaccinations protect both you and your baby — either by protecting you from infections that could harm the pregnancy, or by transferring antibodies through the placenta that will protect your baby in the first weeks of life before their own immune system is mature enough to respond to vaccines.

Vaccinations given routinely in pregnancy:

- Tetanus-diphtheria-pertussis (Tdap): Recommended in every pregnancy, ideally between 27 and 36 weeks. Whooping cough (pertussis) can be fatal in young infants before they are old enough to be immunised. Maternal Tdap vaccination transfers high levels of pertussis antibodies to the baby through the placenta, protecting them in the first 2 to 3 months of life. Under India's national immunisation programme, tetanus toxoid (TT) is given to all pregnant women; Tdap is the preferred option where available.
- Influenza (inactivated): Safe and recommended in any trimester, particularly during influenza season. Pregnant women are at higher risk of severe influenza complications (pneumonia, ICU admission, preterm birth). Inactivated influenza vaccine — the standard injected vaccine — is safe. The live attenuated intranasal vaccine should be avoided in pregnancy.
- COVID-19 (mRNA vaccines): Recommended for pregnant women by WHO, FOGSI, CDC, and all major obstetric bodies. The benefits — protection against severe maternal COVID-19 and its associated preterm birth risk — substantially outweigh the risks, for which extensive safety data now exists from millions of vaccinated pregnancies.

Vaccinations to avoid in pregnancy (live vaccines):

- MMR (measles-mumps-rubella): Live attenuated vaccine. Contraindicated in pregnancy. Administer postpartum if immunity is absent; avoid conception for one month after vaccination.

- Varicella (chickenpox): Live attenuated vaccine. Contraindicated in pregnancy. Varicella infection in the first trimester can cause fetal varicella syndrome (limb defects, eye damage, brain damage); near term it can cause severe neonatal varicella. If a non-immune pregnant woman is exposed to varicella, VZIG (varicella zoster immune globulin) can be given within 96 hours.
- BCG: Avoid in pregnancy.

Your Pregnancy, Your Body, Your Rights

Before we close, I want to say something that is less medical and more human.

Pregnancy in India often involves a great deal of advice. From family, from in-laws, from neighbours, from people you have never met who feel entitled to comment on your body, your choices, and your plans. Some of this advice is kind and useful. Some of it is well-meaning but wrong. Some of it is intrusive and unwelcome.

You have the right to make your own medical decisions. You have the right to be informed — fully, honestly, without condescension — about your options. You have the right to ask questions and to receive answers in language you can understand. You have the right to a second opinion. You have the right to refuse interventions you do not want (with the exception of emergency situations where your life or your baby's life is in immediate danger). You have the right to be treated with dignity and respect in every healthcare encounter.

India has made remarkable progress in maternal health over the past two decades. But we still have much to do — in access, in quality, and in the fundamental respect for pregnant women as autonomous adults capable of making informed decisions about their own bodies and their own care.

Be your own advocate. Ask questions. Do not accept dismissal. If you are not satisfied with the information or the treatment you receive, seek another opinion. And wherever possible, choose a doctor — and a hospital — where you feel genuinely heard.

When to Call Your Doctor

Keep this page somewhere accessible. Show it to your family members too.

GO TO HOSPITAL IMMEDIATELY

- Heavy vaginal bleeding at any stage of pregnancy (soaking more than one pad)
- Severe, one-sided lower abdominal pain in the first trimester (possible ectopic pregnancy)
- Reduced or absent fetal movements after 24 weeks
- Severe headache not responding to paracetamol
- Visual disturbances — flashing lights, blurring, loss of vision
- Upper right abdominal pain or pain under the ribs (liver sign)
- Sudden significant swelling of the face or hands
- Fever above 38°C
- Inability to keep any fluid down for more than 12-24 hours
- Regular contractions before 37 weeks
- Gush or continuous trickle of clear fluid from the vagina
- Anything that makes you feel seriously unwell in a way you cannot explain

Your Antenatal Schedule at a Glance

Visit	When	What Happens
Booking visit	8-10 weeks	Full history, examination, booking blood tests, dating ultrasound
NT scan + blood test	11+0 to 13+6 weeks	Combined first trimester screen, fetal heartbeat and anatomy check
NIPT (optional)	10+ weeks	Cell-free fetal DNA screening for chromosomal conditions
Anomaly scan	18-22 weeks	Detailed fetal anatomy survey, placenta and fluid assessment
Glucose tolerance test	24-28 weeks	75g OGTT — screening for gestational diabetes
Anaemia recheck	28 weeks	FBC, anti-D injection if Rh negative
Growth scan	28-34 weeks	For women with risk factors for fetal growth restriction
GBS swab	35-37 weeks	Group B Streptococcus screening (where offered)
Tdap vaccine	27-36 weeks	Whooping cough protection for baby
Fetal position check	36 weeks	Confirm cephalic presentation; discuss birth plan; ECV if breech
Weekly visits	37-40+ weeks	BP, urine, fetal wellbeing, membrane sweep offered from 39 weeks
Induction review	41 weeks	Induction of labour discussion; electronic fetal monitoring

10

Your Body, Week by Week

What Is Happening Inside You at Every Stage

Every pregnancy book tells you about your baby's development week by week. But your body is also undergoing one of the most extraordinary biological transformations in nature — and it deserves the same detailed attention. This chapter traces the changes in your own body from the first weeks of pregnancy through to the end — the hormonal, cardiovascular, musculoskeletal, dermatological, and neurological shifts that together constitute the maternal adaptation to pregnancy.

Understanding these changes will help you make sense of the symptoms you experience, explain why certain things feel different, and give you a framework for knowing what is normal and what deserves a call to your doctor. Your body is not failing when it produces these changes. It is succeeding — performing a biological task of remarkable complexity.

The First Trimester: Revolution at the Cellular Level

Your Hormones

The first trimester is the most hormonally volatile period of pregnancy. Within days of implantation, hCG — human chorionic gonadotrophin — begins rising, doubling every 48 hours, reaching its peak at approximately 8 to 10 weeks before gradually declining. hCG is the hormone that pregnancy tests detect, and it is the primary driver of the first trimester's most characteristic symptom: nausea.

Progesterone, produced first by the corpus luteum and then increasingly by the placenta from around week 8, rises substantially throughout the first trimester. Progesterone is the pregnancy's main sustaining hormone: it prevents uterine contractions, suppresses the immune response that might otherwise reject the embryo, and prepares the breast tissue for lactation. Its sedative effect on smooth muscle is responsible for many first-trimester symptoms — the constipation (slowed gut motility), the heartburn (relaxed lower oesophageal sphincter), the frequent urination (relaxed bladder), and the profound fatigue (its central sedating effect).

Oestrogen — primarily oestradiol and oestriol, produced by the placenta — also begins rising from early pregnancy. Oestrogen stimulates uterine growth, increases blood volume, promotes breast tissue development, and modulates the effects of progesterone throughout the pregnancy.

Relaxin, produced by the corpus luteum and placenta, begins rising in the first trimester. Its primary role is to loosen the ligaments and cartilage of the pelvic girdle, creating the flexibility needed for birth. Unfortunately, relaxin affects all ligaments, not just pelvic ones — contributing to the joint laxity, back pain, and general physical instability that many women notice from the first trimester onwards.

Human placental lactogen (hPL), produced by the placenta from about week 6, begins its long rise. hPL has insulin-antagonistic effects — it reduces maternal sensitivity to insulin, effectively routing glucose to the fetus. This is the beginning of the progressive insulin resistance of pregnancy that, in susceptible women, leads to gestational diabetes.

Your Blood and Circulation

Blood volume increases dramatically in pregnancy — ultimately rising by 40 to 50% above non-pregnant values. This expansion begins in the first trimester and accelerates throughout. The plasma (liquid) component increases more than the red blood cell component, creating a dilutional anaemia — the haematocrit (percentage of red blood cells in the blood) falls even in women who are not iron-deficient, simply because the plasma has expanded more than the red cell mass. This physiological anaemia is normal and requires no treatment; it is distinguished from true iron-deficiency anaemia by the blood film and iron studies.

The heart's output — the volume of blood pumped per minute — increases by 30 to 50% during pregnancy, beginning in the first trimester. This is achieved by both an increased heart rate (the resting heart rate rises by 10 to 15 beats per minute from early pregnancy) and an increased stroke volume (the amount of blood pumped with each beat). You may notice your heart racing or pounding occasionally — this is physiological in the absence of other symptoms.

Blood pressure falls in the first and second trimesters, reaching its nadir at approximately 20 to 22 weeks, before rising again in the third trimester. This fall is caused by progesterone-mediated vasodilation — the blood vessels relax and widen, reducing the resistance against which the heart pumps. The consequence: many women feel lightheaded, particularly when standing up quickly (orthostatic hypotension). Drink plenty of water, avoid prolonged standing, and rise slowly. This is not dangerous — but it is uncomfortable and sometimes alarming.

Your Immune System

Pregnancy requires a fundamental modification of the immune system. The fetus is, immunologically speaking, foreign tissue — it carries the father's antigens as well as the mother's. For the pregnancy to continue, the maternal immune system must be selectively suppressed at the placental interface, preventing rejection of the fetus while maintaining adequate immune function against genuine infections.

This is achieved through a complex set of immunological adaptations: increased regulatory T-cell activity at the placental site, altered cytokine balance (a shift from Th1 to Th2 immune responses), and local immune suppression by placental factors. The practical consequence: some autoimmune conditions (rheumatoid arthritis, multiple sclerosis) improve during pregnancy, because the immune suppression reduces the autoimmune attack. Others (systemic lupus erythematosus) can flare. Infections that are managed normally outside of pregnancy — particularly viral infections such as influenza, varicella, and COVID-19 — can be more severe in pregnant women.

Your Kidneys

Renal blood flow increases by 40 to 60% in pregnancy, and glomerular filtration rate (the kidney's filtering rate) increases by a similar amount. This increased filtration explains several first-trimester phenomena: the increased urinary frequency (more urine is being produced), the lower blood creatinine (the kidney filters it more efficiently — a normal creatinine of 70 micromol/L in a non-pregnant woman might be 50 in a pregnant woman), and the occasional presence of glucose in the urine without gestational diabetes (the increased filtering can overwhelm the kidney's reabsorption capacity for glucose).

The ureters (tubes connecting the kidneys to the bladder) dilate in pregnancy under the influence of progesterone and mechanical compression from the growing uterus. This dilation slows urinary flow and creates stasis — standing pools of urine in the dilated ureters — that provide an excellent culture medium for bacteria. This is why asymptomatic bacteriuria (bacteria in the urine without symptoms) is screened for at the booking visit: if left untreated, it progresses to symptomatic urinary tract infection and pyelonephritis (kidney infection) in approximately 25 to 30% of affected pregnant women, with significant preterm labour risk.

The Second Trimester: A Body Transformed

The Uterus

The uterus undergoes one of the most extraordinary organ transformations in biology. Before pregnancy, it weighs approximately 50 to 70 grams and has a capacity of about 10 mL. At term, it weighs approximately 1,000 grams (a 14-fold increase) and has a capacity of 5,000 to 10,000 mL. This growth is achieved through hypertrophy of existing muscle fibres (each smooth muscle cell increasing to approximately 500 times its non-pregnant volume) and hyperplasia (new cell formation), driven by oestrogen and mechanical stretch.

The fundal height — the distance from the pubic symphysis to the top of the uterus — increases by approximately 1 centimetre per week from 20 weeks onwards. At 20 weeks, the fundus reaches the umbilicus. At 36 weeks, it reaches the xiphisternum (the lower end of the breastbone). After engagement of the fetal head at 36 to 38 weeks in primigravid women, the fundus may drop slightly as the baby descends into the pelvis.

Braxton-Hicks contractions — irregular, painless tightenings of the uterus — begin as early as 6 to 7 weeks but are typically not felt until the second trimester. They represent practice contractions: the uterine muscle warming up for the sustained, coordinated work of labour. They become more frequent and noticeable as pregnancy advances, particularly in the third trimester. Their distinguishing feature from true labour contractions is their irregularity and their tendency to ease with rest, hydration, or position change.

Your Skin

The skin of pregnancy is a visible record of the hormonal changes occurring within. Oestrogen, progesterone, and melanocyte-stimulating hormone (MSH) all affect skin pigmentation, vascularity, and texture.

Linea nigra — the dark line running from the pubic symphysis to the umbilicus (and often beyond) — appears in the majority of women during the second trimester. It represents hyperpigmentation along the embryological fusion line of the two halves of the abdomen. It is entirely benign and fades, though rarely disappears completely, after delivery.

Chloasma (melasma, or the "mask of pregnancy") — irregular patches of hyperpigmentation on the face, particularly the cheeks, forehead, upper lip, and around the eyes — affects approximately 50 to 70% of pregnant women. It is caused by increased MSH stimulating melanocytes. It is exacerbated by sun exposure — use SPF 30 or higher sunscreen daily if you are prone to it. It fades after delivery but may take many months and sometimes does not fully resolve.

Spider naevi — small, spider-shaped vascular lesions on the face, neck, upper chest, and arms — appear due to oestrogen-induced capillary dilation. Most resolve after delivery. Palmar erythema — reddening of the palms — has the same cause.

Increased sweating and heat intolerance: The 40 to 50% increase in blood volume means the body must dissipate significantly more heat. Sweating increases, and many women feel uncomfortably hot, particularly in the third trimester. This is normal — wear breathable natural fabrics, keep environments cool, and stay well hydrated.

Nail and hair changes: Many women notice their hair becomes thicker and faster-growing during pregnancy — oestrogen prolongs the growth phase of the hair cycle, preventing the normal daily shedding. The inevitable consequence: postpartum, when oestrogen falls, large amounts of hair are shed simultaneously. Postpartum alopecia — significant hair loss beginning at 3 to 6 months after delivery — affects the majority of women and is caused by this synchronised shedding of telogen (resting phase) hairs. It is alarming. It is temporary. It completely resolves by 12 months postpartum in almost all women.

Your Breasts

Breast changes are among the earliest and most consistent signs of pregnancy. Under the influence of oestrogen, progesterone, prolactin, and hPL, the breast undergoes dramatic remodelling throughout pregnancy.

In the first trimester: tenderness, heaviness, and tingling — the result of rapid ductal proliferation and increased blood flow. The areolae darken and enlarge. Montgomery's tubercles — the small bumps around the areola that secrete lubricating fluid — become more prominent. Superficial veins become visible on the breast skin.

In the second trimester: the breasts increase significantly in size as lobular development accelerates. Colostrum — the first milk — may begin to leak in small amounts from as early as the second trimester. This is not a problem; it is simply early evidence of lactogenesis. Use breast pads if the leaking is inconvenient.

By the third trimester, the breasts have completed their structural preparation for lactation and may be producing colostrum regularly. The breast size increase across pregnancy is typically one to two cup sizes — with the implication that your bra size will need reassessment, ideally by a trained fitter.

Your Musculoskeletal System

The musculoskeletal changes of pregnancy are among the most practically significant for daily life. The growing uterus progressively shifts the centre of gravity forward, compensating for which requires an increasing lumbar lordosis (inward curve of the lower back). This postural adaptation, combined with relaxin-mediated ligamentous laxity, creates the characteristic gait of late pregnancy and the very common complaint of lower back pain.

The pelvic girdle — comprising the sacroiliac joints and the pubic symphysis — undergoes deliberate loosening under the influence of relaxin, creating the pelvic flexibility needed for birth. In most women, this is asymptomatic or mildly uncomfortable. In approximately 20% of women, it causes significant pelvic girdle pain (PGP): pain at the pubic symphysis, the sacroiliac joints, or both, that can range from an ache to severe disability.

The carpal tunnel syndrome of pregnancy — numbness, tingling, and pain in the thumb, index, and middle fingers, worst at night — results from fluid retention compressing the median nerve within the carpal tunnel at the wrist. It affects approximately 20 to 35% of pregnant women and typically begins in the second trimester, worsening in the third. Management: wrist splints worn at night, elevation of the hands, reduction of repetitive wrist movements. It almost always resolves completely after delivery.

Leg cramps — sudden, severe painful cramps in the calf muscles, typically occurring at night — affect approximately 30 to 50% of pregnant women, most commonly in the third trimester. Their exact cause is uncertain; magnesium deficiency, reduced venous return from the legs, and nerve compression are all implicated. Management: regular calf stretching before bed, adequate magnesium intake (nuts, seeds, leafy greens, dark chocolate), and dorsiflexion of the foot (pulling the toes toward the shin) during an acute cramp.

The Third Trimester: Final Preparations

Breathing and the Diaphragm

As the uterus grows into the upper abdomen, it progressively elevates the diaphragm — the dome-shaped muscle that separates the chest from the abdomen. By 36 weeks, the diaphragm has been pushed upward by approximately 4 centimetres. The chest compensates by expanding outward — the transverse diameter of the chest increases by approximately 2 centimetres, and the rib flare that many women notice in the third trimester is this expansion.

The practical consequence: breathlessness. The lungs have less space to expand downward, and the increased oxygen demand of the pregnant body (basal metabolic rate increases by 15 to 20%) means every breath is working harder. Physiological breathlessness in the third trimester is normal. Breathlessness that is severe, sudden, associated with chest pain, or accompanied by a faster heart rate requires urgent assessment — pulmonary embolism and peripartum cardiomyopathy must be excluded.

At approximately 36 to 38 weeks in first-time mothers, the baby's head engages in the pelvis — "lightening" occurs. The top of the uterus drops away from the diaphragm, and breathing suddenly becomes easier. The trade-off: the pelvis is now under more pressure, and walking becomes waddling.

Oedema — Swelling

Physiological oedema — swelling of the ankles, feet, and sometimes hands — affects approximately 80% of pregnant women in the third trimester. It is caused by the increased venous pressure in the lower limbs (from the weight of the pregnant uterus on the pelvic veins), reduced plasma oncotic pressure (the dilutional effect of the expanded plasma volume), and increased capillary permeability mediated by pregnancy hormones.

Physiological oedema is worse at the end of the day, in hot weather, after prolonged standing, and in the third trimester. It is symmetrical (affecting both ankles equally), is not associated with high blood pressure or protein in the urine, and improves dramatically after lying down (particularly on the left side, which relieves the inferior vena cava compression) or elevating the legs.

It is distinguished from pathological oedema (associated with pre-eclampsia) by the absence of hypertension and proteinuria, and by its non-facial distribution — oedema of the face, particularly on waking, is more concerning and warrants blood pressure measurement.

Management of physiological oedema: graduated compression stockings (wear from first thing in the morning, before any swelling begins), regular elevation of the legs, avoiding prolonged standing, regular walking (calf muscle contractions act as a venous pump), and staying well hydrated. Reducing salt modestly is sensible, but severe sodium restriction is not recommended in pregnancy.

Sleep

Sleep in the third trimester is disrupted by multiple converging factors: physical discomfort (finding a comfortable position with a large bump is a project in itself), frequent urination (nocturia), leg cramps, vivid and sometimes disturbing dreams (progesterone's effect on sleep architecture), restless legs syndrome (associated with iron and folate deficiency), fetal movements at inconvenient hours, and the mental activity of an approaching major life event.

Restless legs syndrome (RLS) — an uncontrollable urge to move the legs, particularly at night, associated with uncomfortable sensations described as crawling, tingling, or throbbing — affects approximately 26% of pregnant women, with a peak in the third trimester. It is strongly associated with iron-deficiency anaemia (even borderline anaemia) and folate deficiency. Treatment: ensure adequate iron and folate status; gentle exercise during the day; warm baths before bed; magnesium supplementation.

Positioning for sleep: The left lateral position is recommended from 28 weeks onwards to reduce compression of the inferior vena cava by the uterus, which can reduce blood return to the heart. A pillow between the knees, another supporting the abdomen, and one behind the back ("a pillow nest") significantly improves comfort. Specially shaped pregnancy pillows (C-shape or U-shape) are widely available and genuinely helpful for many women. If you wake up on your back, simply roll to your side. Lying briefly on your back will not harm your baby — but sustained supine position (particularly if it causes you to feel faint or nauseous) should be avoided.

Labour: Your Body at its Most Powerful

Cervical Ripening

In the final weeks before labour, the cervix undergoes a process called ripening — a transformation from a firm, closed, posterior-pointing structure to a soft, effaced (thinned), dilated, anterior-pointing one. This process is driven by prostaglandins and inflammatory mediators that degrade the collagen fibres that give the cervix its firmness, and by increasing hyaluronic acid that absorbs water and softens the tissue.

Cervical ripeness is assessed using the Bishop score — a scoring system based on five parameters: dilation, effacement, station (how far the baby's head has descended), consistency, and position of the cervix. A Bishop score above 6 indicates a ripe, favourable cervix likely to respond well to induction of labour; a score below 6 indicates an unfavourable cervix that may need ripening agents before induction is likely to succeed.

The Pelvic Floor

The pelvic floor — the hammock of muscles, ligaments, and fascia that spans the base of the pelvis — is one of the most remarkable and most neglected structures in the female body. It supports the uterus, bladder, and rectum; maintains continence of urine and faeces; plays an important role in sexual function; and, at birth, must stretch to accommodate the passage of the baby's head — typically 10 centimetres in diameter.

The pelvic floor's ability to stretch to this degree and then recover is extraordinary — but not unconditional. Prolonged second stage of labour, instrumental delivery (forceps or vacuum), large babies, multiple pregnancies, and inadequate pelvic floor rehabilitation after birth all increase the risk of long-term pelvic floor dysfunction: stress urinary incontinence, pelvic organ prolapse, and dyspareunia (painful intercourse).

The evidence for pelvic floor exercises (Kegel exercises) in pregnancy and the postpartum period is robust: regular pelvic floor training reduces the risk of urinary incontinence in pregnancy and after birth, promotes faster recovery of pelvic floor function, and reduces the risk of prolapse. They should be started as early as possible in pregnancy and continued for life.

How to do them correctly: First, identify the correct muscles. The next time you urinate, try to stop the flow mid-stream. The muscles you use are your pelvic floor. (Do this as a test only — do not practise stopping urine flow regularly, as this disrupts the normal voiding reflex.) Contract these muscles, hold for 5 to 10 seconds, then relax completely — the relaxation is as important as the contraction. Repeat 10 times, three sets daily. Add quick flicks — rapid contractions and releases — for additional benefit. Do them sitting, lying, standing. Do them in the queue at the vegetable market. No one will know.

✍ My NOTE

The pelvic floor is the most important structure you have never been taught about. I spend approximately five minutes at every booking visit talking about pelvic floor exercises, and approximately five minutes at every postnatal check asking whether women are doing them. The answer is usually no. I understand — with a newborn, pelvic floor exercises feel absurdly low priority. But incontinence, which affects approximately one in three women who have given birth, is not inevitable. It is largely preventable. The five minutes a day you invest in your pelvic floor before and after birth will pay dividends for the rest of your life.

11

Moving Your Body

Exercise, Yoga, and Rest Throughout Pregnancy

There is a persistent mythology around exercise in pregnancy — that rest is protective, that exertion is risky, that the cautious woman keeps herself still and safe. This mythology, well-intentioned though it may be, has caused genuine harm. The evidence, accumulated over decades of rigorous research, says something different: regular moderate exercise throughout a healthy pregnancy is not only safe — it is one of the most beneficial things you can do for yourself and your baby.

What the Evidence Says

The benefits of exercise in pregnancy are substantial and well-documented:

- Reduces the risk of gestational diabetes by 30 to 38% — one of the strongest preventive interventions available for this increasingly common condition
- Reduces the risk of pre-eclampsia by approximately 35%
- Limits excessive gestational weight gain
- Reduces lower back pain and pelvic girdle pain — not because exercise prevents the underlying ligamentous laxity, but because strengthened core and hip muscles better support the destabilised pelvis
- Reduces symptoms of depression and anxiety in pregnancy — robust evidence from multiple randomised controlled trials
- Reduces the risk of caesarean section and operative vaginal delivery
- Shortens the duration of labour in several studies
- Reduces the risk of macrosomia (very large baby) — partly by reducing gestational diabetes risk
- Improves sleep quality
- Speeds postpartum recovery

The guidelines from ACOG, RCOG, and FOGSI are consistent: women with uncomplicated pregnancies should aim for at least 150 minutes of moderate-intensity aerobic activity per week, in bouts of at least 10 minutes. This equates to 30 minutes on five days of the week, or 50 minutes on three days. This is the same recommendation as for non-pregnant adults — pregnancy does not reduce the need for physical activity; if anything, the benefits are amplified.

What Is Safe: Trimester by Trimester

First Trimester

If you were active before pregnancy, continue your activities with minor modifications. If you were sedentary, start gradually — 10 to 15 minutes of walking daily, increasing toward 30 minutes as your body adapts. The first trimester is the period of greatest fatigue and nausea, and "exercise" may feel like a distant aspiration when you cannot eat without feeling sick. That is acceptable. Do what you can.

Avoid: hot yoga and Bikram yoga (core temperature above 38.9°C is potentially harmful to the embryo in the first trimester, particularly during the critical period of neural tube closure and organogenesis); very high-intensity exercise that takes your heart rate to maximum and leaves you unable to speak (the "talk test" — if you can carry on a conversation while exercising, the intensity is appropriate); anything with a high fall risk if you are not accustomed to it.

Safe and recommended: walking, swimming, cycling (stationary or outdoor on flat terrain), prenatal yoga (with appropriate modifications), light to moderate strength training.

Second Trimester

The second trimester is usually the easiest for exercise — nausea has typically passed, energy has returned, and the bump is not yet large enough to significantly impair movement. This is the trimester in which to establish a regular exercise habit if you have not done so already.

From approximately 20 weeks, avoid exercises that require lying flat on your back for prolonged periods — the uterus can compress the inferior vena cava in this position, reducing blood return to the heart and potentially causing supine hypotensive syndrome. This does not mean you can never lie on your back for a brief stretch; it means you should not hold static supine positions for extended periods in yoga, Pilates, or core exercises.

Core exercises: The core changes significantly in pregnancy. As the uterus grows and the rectus abdominis muscles (the "six-pack") separate to accommodate it — a process called diastasis recti — traditional core exercises such as sit-ups and crunches become contraindicated from the second trimester onwards. They increase intra-abdominal pressure in a way that can worsen the diastasis and stress the pelvic floor. Replace them with pelvic tilts, cat-cow stretches, bird-dog exercises, side planks, and deep breathing with engagement of the transverse abdominis (the deep core muscle that is the foundation of functional core strength).

Third Trimester

The third trimester requires adaptations to exercise for practical reasons: the bump alters your centre of gravity and your range of motion, balance is affected, and the added weight of pregnancy makes activities that were previously easy feel significantly harder. The goal shifts from performance or intensity toward maintenance and mobility.

Walking remains ideal throughout the third trimester — even a gentle 20-minute walk daily maintains cardiovascular fitness, promotes fetal engagement, reduces oedema, and provides the psychological benefit of movement and fresh air. Swimming and water aerobics become particularly valuable as the buoyancy of water supports the weight of the bump, relieves joint pressure, and allows movements that are difficult on land.

Avoid: exercises that involve lying on the back for sustained periods; contact sports; activities with high fall risk (cycling outdoors becomes less safe as balance is affected); scuba diving (the fetus cannot decompress safely); exercise at high altitude above 2,500 metres if unacclimatised.

Absolute Contraindications to Exercise in Pregnancy

The following conditions require cessation of aerobic exercise and consultation with your doctor:

- Haemodynamically significant heart or lung disease
- Cervical insufficiency or cerclage (a stitch in the cervix)
- Active preterm labour
- Placenta praevia after 26 weeks
- Severe anaemia (haemoglobin below 8 g/dL)
- Poorly controlled hypertension or pre-eclampsia
- Poorly controlled type 1 diabetes, thyroid disease, or seizure disorder
- Rupture of membranes (once waters have broken, exercise is inappropriate)

Stop Exercising and Call Your Doctor if You Experience:

- Vaginal bleeding
- Dizziness or fainting
- Chest pain or palpitations
- Difficulty breathing beyond normal exercise breathlessness
- Calf pain or swelling (possible DVT)
- Regular uterine contractions
- Leaking of fluid
- Decreased fetal movements
- Headache or visual disturbances during exercise

Yoga in Pregnancy

Prenatal yoga has accumulated impressive evidence for its benefits across all three trimesters. Randomised controlled trials have demonstrated: reduced rates of preterm birth, lower perceived pain scores in labour, shorter first stage of labour, lower rates of operative delivery, reduced antenatal anxiety and depression, and improved maternal sleep quality. These are not trivial effects — they represent outcomes that matter clinically.

Yoga's benefits in pregnancy are mediated through multiple pathways: the physical strengthening of muscles used in labour (gluteals, pelvic floor, core); the cultivation of breath awareness and controlled breathing that is directly applicable to managing labour contractions; the reduction of cortisol through the relaxation response; and the mental discipline of remaining present and calm in a situation of physical intensity — exactly the skill required in labour.

Modifications for Pregnancy

Not all yoga poses are appropriate in pregnancy. The following modifications are important:

Avoid deep forward bends in which the abdomen is compressed — as the uterus grows, this becomes both uncomfortable and potentially problematic. Widen the stance in forward bends to create space for the belly.

Avoid deep twists that rotate from the waist — these compress the uterus and placenta. Replace with open twists that rotate from the upper chest and shoulders only, creating space in the abdomen rather than compressing it.

Avoid all poses involving lying flat on the back from the second trimester — replace with side-lying alternatives or bolstered modifications.

Avoid inversions (headstand, shoulderstand, handstand) unless you are highly experienced in these poses and have your teacher's guidance — the fall risk and the risk of air entering the uterine veins in the inverted position both justify caution.

Avoid hot yoga and Bikram yoga — as discussed, hyperthermia is genuinely harmful in pregnancy.

Avoid lying prone (on the stomach) from the second trimester onwards.

Particularly valuable poses: Cat-cow (marjaryasana-bitilasana) for back pain and spinal mobility; squatting (malasana) for pelvic floor lengthening and hip opening — highly valuable preparation for birth; child's pose (balasana, with knees wide for the belly) for rest and back release; warrior II (virabhadrasana II) for strength and grounding; side-lying savasana for deep relaxation.

My NOTE

I recommend prenatal yoga to virtually all my patients. Not because I am a yoga enthusiast (I am a moderately flexible obstetrician who falls out of tree pose more often than I would like to admit), but because the evidence is clear and because I have seen, over many years, that women who practise yoga in pregnancy tend to approach labour with a quality of readiness — both physical and psychological — that is genuinely different from those who have not. They know how to breathe through intensity. They have practised being calm when something is uncomfortable. These are not small skills in labour.

Swimming and Water Exercise

Swimming is perhaps the ideal pregnancy exercise. The buoyancy of water supports the weight of the uterus and growing baby, eliminating the musculoskeletal stress that makes most land-based exercise progressively more challenging in the third trimester. Water resistance provides a gentle but effective cardiovascular and strength workout without impact. The horizontal position in water relieves the postural strain that upright positions impose. And many women find the sensation of weightlessness in water — after weeks of carrying a substantial bump — deeply restorative.

Breaststroke can aggravate pelvic girdle pain because of the asymmetric hip movement — if you experience PGP, prefer front crawl or backstroke, or consider water walking in the shallow end. Avoid diving and jumping into the water, particularly in the second and third trimesters. Swimming pools should be chlorinated, not hot tubs — water temperature above 35°C is not appropriate for prolonged immersion in pregnancy.

Walking: Underrated and Brilliant

Walking is the most accessible, most sustainable, and most universally applicable exercise of pregnancy. It requires no equipment, no gym membership, no special training. It can be done at any intensity, any duration, and at any gestational age. It can be done in the early morning in your neighbourhood, on a treadmill at your office, or in the evening with your partner. It can be done in a sari.

30 minutes of brisk walking daily — brisk meaning a pace at which you can speak but not sing — provides significant cardiovascular benefit, helps control gestational weight gain, reduces the risk of gestational diabetes, promotes fetal descent in the third trimester, and provides the well-established mental health benefits of regular physical activity combined with outdoor exposure.

If nausea prevents morning exercise in the first trimester, walk in the evening when nausea often eases. If the heat is prohibitive in Indian summers, walk early in the morning or after dark. If swelling makes walking uncomfortable in the third trimester, wear compression stockings and comfortable, supportive footwear. There is almost always a way.

Pelvic Floor Exercises: The Non-Negotiable

Pelvic floor exercises are not optional. They are not something to fit in when you remember. They are one of the most evidence-based preventive interventions available to every pregnant woman, and they deserve to be treated with the same seriousness as taking your iron supplement.

Stress urinary incontinence — leaking urine when coughing, sneezing, laughing, or jumping — affects approximately 30 to 40% of women in the third trimester and approximately 33% of women one year after their first vaginal birth. It is not inevitable, and it is not something you simply have to accept as the price of motherhood. Regular pelvic floor training in pregnancy significantly reduces its occurrence, and postnatal pelvic floor rehabilitation restores continence in the majority of affected women.

The routine: 10 slow contractions held for 10 seconds, followed by 10 quick flicks, three times daily. This takes approximately 5 minutes. Do it when you wake up. Do it during your lunch break. Do it before you go to sleep. Tie it to something you already do: every time you brew chai, every time you sit in a traffic jam, every time a meeting runs over schedule.

Rest: The Other Side of the Equation

Exercise is important. So is rest. And in India, where the cultural expectation is often that a pregnant woman continues every aspect of her role — working, cooking, managing the household, attending social obligations — until labour begins, the permission to rest is sometimes the most important thing a doctor can give.

Fatigue in pregnancy is not laziness. It is a physiological signal. The profound first-trimester fatigue is your body redirecting energy resources toward the extraordinary task of building a placenta and an embryo simultaneously. The third-trimester exhaustion is the consequence of carrying an additional 10 to 15 kilograms, sleeping poorly, and approaching a major physical event. Both are legitimate reasons to rest.

Practical rest strategies: Lie down for 20 to 30 minutes in the afternoon if at all possible — even in the second trimester when energy has largely returned. A brief rest in the afternoon dramatically reduces evening fatigue and improves sleep quality. Delegate tasks that do not need to be done by you. Accept offers of help without guilt. Reduce non-essential social commitments, particularly in the third trimester. Sleep as much as your body asks for in the first trimester — 9 to 10 hours is not unusual and is completely appropriate.

" Geeta's Running

"My mother-in-law told me I should stop going to the gym from the moment I got pregnant," Geeta said, frustrated. "My colleagues keep telling me to sit down. My husband wants me to take a taxi for everything. I am 14 weeks pregnant, not an invalid." She was a regular runner — 5 kilometres three times a week before pregnancy. I told her: continue. Run at a pace where you can maintain a conversation. Reduce intensity if you feel breathless or uncomfortable. Stop if you bleed, have contractions, or feel unwell. Listen to your body — not to people who are not obstetricians. She ran until 28 weeks, then switched to swimming. She delivered at 39+2, had a four-hour active labour, and was walking to the local chai shop the next day. "I think running helped," she told me. I told her: I think so too.

12

Your Relationships and Emotional Life

Navigating Pregnancy with the People You Love

Pregnancy does not happen in isolation. It happens inside a family, a relationship, a social world — full of people with opinions, expectations, histories, and their own complicated feelings about the arrival of a new baby. Navigating all of this while also growing a human being is its own significant project.

This chapter is about the relational and emotional landscape of pregnancy: your relationship with your partner, the complex dynamics of extended family (particularly in the Indian joint family context), the particular challenges of the workplace, and the emotional work of becoming a mother.

Your Relationship with Your Partner

Pregnancy is often described as bringing couples closer. And sometimes it does — the shared experience of anticipating a child, the first scan, the moment of quickening, the gradual building of a new identity as parents. These experiences can be profoundly bonding.

But pregnancy also introduces strains that are rarely talked about honestly: the physical changes that make sex different or difficult or unwanted; the emotional asymmetry of carrying a pregnancy (you are living it from the inside; your partner is witnessing it from the outside); the financial pressures that a new child intensifies; the disagreements about parenting philosophy that begin, sometimes surprisingly, before the baby is even born.

Intimacy and Sex During Pregnancy

Sex during pregnancy is safe for the vast majority of women, throughout the entire pregnancy, in the absence of specific medical contraindications. These contraindications include: placenta praevia (where penile penetration or orgasm could trigger bleeding), cervical insufficiency or cerclage, unexplained vaginal bleeding, preterm labour, or ruptured membranes. In the presence of any of these conditions, abstain from penetrative intercourse and discuss with your doctor what sexual activity is and is not appropriate.

For everyone else: the baby is protected within the amniotic sac, surrounded by fluid, sealed off from the vagina by the mucous plug in the cervix. Penetrative intercourse cannot harm the baby. Orgasm causes uterine contractions, but these are entirely different from labour contractions and will not initiate labour in a healthy pregnancy at term.

That said, desire changes. In the first trimester, nausea, fatigue, and breast tenderness conspire to make many women entirely disinterested in sex — and this is completely normal. In the second trimester, increased pelvic blood flow, improved energy, and the extraordinary experience of feeling connected to your own body in a new way lead many women to experience increased sexual interest. In the third trimester, physical discomfort — the bump, the back pain, the awkwardness of finding a comfortable position — often reduces desire again, though this is variable.

Positions: From approximately 20 weeks, women on top positions accommodate the bump and are generally most comfortable. Communication with your partner about what is and is not comfortable is, of course, essential.

For partners: understand that a woman whose body is working this hard, who may feel nauseated and exhausted and physically inhabited in a new and sometimes overwhelming way, may have very different feelings about physical intimacy than usual. This is not rejection. This is pregnancy. Patience, physical affection that is not always sexual, and explicit reassurance that intimacy is not exclusively about sex ,these matter.

Communicating Your Needs

One of the most common patterns I observe in couples during pregnancy is a gradual accumulation of unspoken needs. The pregnant woman does not want to seem demanding; her partner does not want to say the wrong thing; and so the things that most need to be said — "I need more help at home," "I am frightened about birth and I need you to take it seriously," "I feel invisible in this pregnancy" — go unsaid until they become resentments.

Specific conversations worth having before the third trimester:

- What does support during labour look like to you? What do you need your partner to do, say, or not say? Have you discussed this?
- Who will be present at the birth? Both of you need to agree on this — and cultural expectations (mothers-in-law in the delivery room) should be discussed openly, with your own preferences clearly articulated.
- What will the division of labour look like in the postpartum period? Who takes night feeds? Who handles daytime care? What about household management?
- How will you maintain your relationship as a couple when you are also new parents? When will you have time alone together? How important is this to each of you?

These conversations are uncomfortable because they require honesty about needs, expectations, and differences. Have them anyway. The alternative — figuring it out in the fourth trimester when you are both sleep-deprived and overwhelmed — is significantly worse.

✍ My NOTE

The most common thing I hear from women at their six-week postnatal check, when I ask about their relationship: "He doesn't understand." Sometimes this means the partner is genuinely failing to engage. More often, it means there has been no clear communication — the woman expected him to intuit what she needed, he did not intuit it correctly, and both are hurt and frustrated. Partners are not mind readers. Tell him specifically what you need. "I need you to take the baby from 6 to 9 p.m. every evening so I can shower and have dinner." "I need you to tell me I am doing well, even if everything feels chaotic." Specific requests get results that general expectations do not.

The Extended Family: A Particular Indian Experience

Pregnancy in India is rarely a private affair between two people. It is a family event — sometimes a community event — in which grandmothers, aunts, mothers-in-law, and neighbours all have stakes, opinions, and traditional practices to offer. This involvement is, at its best, a profound support system. At its most challenging, it is a source of conflicting advice, unwanted interventions, and the particular exhaustion of managing other people's emotions about your pregnancy while managing your own.

The volume of advice directed at pregnant women in India is extraordinary. Much of it is well-intentioned and harmless. Some of it is actively wrong and occasionally harmful. The challenge is distinguishing between the two, and doing so without alienating the people who are, after all, expressing their care for you.

A framework that many of my patients find helpful: divide advice into three categories.

Harmless and perhaps pleasant: "Eat ghee every day." "Rest in the afternoons." "Listen to calming music." "Apply oil to your belly." These practices are culturally meaningful, provide the giver with the satisfaction of contributing, and are genuinely not harmful. Smile, thank them, and decide for yourself whether to follow them.

Wrong but low-stakes: "Don't eat papaya." "Don't have your photo taken." "Don't cross your legs." "Sleep with your head facing east." These beliefs, while medically unsupported, are unlikely to affect your pregnancy adversely whether you follow them or not. The question is whether you can tolerate them without significant stress. If yes, nod and move on. If no — if the advice is causing you genuine anxiety or restricting something you value — a gentle, factual clarification may be appropriate.

Potentially harmful: Advice to stop prescribed medication "because it will harm the baby." Advice to fast for extended periods. Advice to use herbal remedies with known uterotonic or teratogenic properties. Advice that is causing you measurable stress. These require a firmer response. "My doctor has advised me on this, and I am following her guidance" is a complete and sufficient answer. You do not need to win the argument; you need to protect yourself and your baby.

The Mother-in-Law Question

In the Indian joint family context, the mother-in-law's role in a pregnancy — and particularly in the postpartum period — is often significant and sometimes overwhelming. Many women receive enormous practical support, emotional comfort, and practical wisdom from their mothers-in-law. Others find the experience of postnatal recovery complicated by a constant presence, traditional practices they do not wish to observe, and the difficulty of asserting their own preferences and boundaries in someone else's home.

A few principles that may help navigate this:

Your partner's role in this negotiation is critical. It is very difficult for you to set limits with your in-laws directly without damaging the relationship. Where possible, let your partner communicate your preferences — "She needs to sleep now," "Her doctor has said she should feed the baby herself," "We have decided to do it this way." This protects your relationship with your in-laws and places the responsibility appropriately on your partner.

Choose your moments of negotiation. You do not need to resist every traditional practice. Decide what matters most to you —

feeding choices, medication decisions, your own physical space and rest — and focus your energy there. Let smaller things go.

Express gratitude for what is genuinely helpful. The acknowledgement of support makes the setting of limits elsewhere feel less confrontational.

Work and Career During Pregnancy

Most women work throughout their pregnancies, often until very close to their due date. This is reasonable, healthy, and for most women, entirely appropriate. But pregnancy does affect your experience of work, and your rights in the workplace deserve to be clearly understood.

Your Legal Rights

The Maternity Benefit (Amendment) Act, 2017 provides the following entitlements to women working in establishments with 10 or more employees:

- 26 weeks of paid maternity leave for the first two children
- 12 weeks of paid maternity leave for the third child onwards
- 12 weeks for women who adopt a child below the age of three months, or for commissioning mothers in surrogacy arrangements
- A break of two nursing breaks of prescribed duration until the child reaches the age of 15 months
- For establishments with 50 or more employees: crèche facilities within a prescribed distance
- The option to work from home (where the nature of work permits) after the maternity leave period, under conditions mutually agreed

You have the right to inform your employer of your pregnancy at a time of your choosing. You are not legally required to disclose your pregnancy before you are ready. Many women wait until after the 12-week scan; others wait longer.

Discrimination based on pregnancy — including termination of employment because of pregnancy, failure to promote, or reduction in salary or responsibilities — is illegal under Indian law and constitutes a violation of the Maternity Benefit Act.

Managing Pregnancy at Work

Practical strategies for working through pregnancy:

First trimester: Nausea and fatigue are the primary challenges. Keep plain crackers and water at your desk. Identify the location of the nearest bathroom. If nausea peaks at a predictable time, plan your heaviest workload for the periods when you feel best. If you need to take sick leave for hyperemesis, it should be recorded as a pregnancy-related illness — it should not be counted against your sickness record in a way that disadvantages you.

Second trimester: Energy typically returns and most women find the second trimester the most productive period of pregnancy. Communicate with your manager or HR department about your pregnancy before your bump becomes obvious — being proactive creates a better dynamic than being caught off-guard. Discuss any necessary adjustments: a chair with better back support, the ability to take brief breaks, adjusted physical duties.

Third trimester: Fatigue returns, commuting becomes more tiring, and concentration may be affected. Plan your maternity leave start date with your doctor's input — most women are advised to stop working at 36 weeks in uncomplicated pregnancies, though many continue longer and this is a personal decision. If you work in a physically demanding role (prolonged standing, heavy lifting, exposure to hazardous substances), earlier leave or modified duties are indicated.

The "maternity leave guilt" is real — the concern about leaving colleagues with extra work, about being perceived as less committed, about the projects that will continue without you. I want to offer a perspective: you are taking leave that you are legally entitled to, for the most important work you will ever do. Prepare your handover thoroughly. Do your job well while you are there. And then leave without guilt.

The Emotional Work of Becoming a Mother

Becoming a mother is not only a physical event. It is a psychological and social transformation — what developmental psychologists call "matrescence," by analogy with adolescence. Just as adolescence is the developmental process of becoming an adult, matrescence is the developmental process of becoming a mother. It involves a profound renegotiation of identity, relationship, and self.

This process is rarely comfortable, and it is almost never linear. You may find yourself cycling through emotions that seem contradictory: fierce love alongside grief for your previous life; profound connection alongside moments of bewildering disconnection; certainty alongside terror; joy alongside exhaustion.

These are not signs that something is wrong with you. They are the signs that something very large is happening. They deserve to be acknowledged — in private, with your partner, with trusted friends, and sometimes with a professional.

Anxiety in Pregnancy

Anxiety is the most common mental health experience of pregnancy — more common than depression, though less discussed. The specific anxieties of pregnancy are real and understandable: fear of miscarriage, particularly in the first trimester or after a previous loss; fear of fetal abnormality; fear of birth; fear of being an inadequate mother; fear of the unknown.

At a moderate level, this anxiety is a normal aspect of the psychological work of pregnancy — the mind preparing for and rehearsing the significant change ahead. It becomes clinically significant when it is disproportionate, persistent, and interfering with daily function: when it prevents sleep, disrupts relationships, causes physical symptoms (palpitations, breathlessness, nausea beyond pregnancy nausea), or is dominated by intrusive, repetitive thoughts that cannot be controlled.

Tokophobia — pathological fear of childbirth — affects approximately 6 to 10% of women. In its primary form (in women who have not previously given birth), it is often rooted in a combination of general anxiety, specific fear of pain or loss of control, and traumatic medical experiences in other contexts. In its secondary form (following a previous difficult birth), it represents a post-traumatic response. Both forms are treatable with skilled psychological support: cognitive behavioural therapy, narrative exposure therapy, and birth planning with a senior clinician who will acknowledge the fears and work with them rather than dismissing them.

If you are experiencing significant anxiety in pregnancy, please tell your doctor. It is not weakness. It is not irrational. It is a clinical condition that has effective treatments, and suffering in silence serves no one.

" Nisha's Fear

"I cannot stop thinking about something going wrong," Nisha told me at 20 weeks. She was healthy, the baby was healthy, the 20-week scan had been normal. "Every time I feel the baby move, I think: what if that's the last time? Every time I have a good day, I think: something bad is about to happen." She paused. "I know I sound crazy." She did not sound crazy. She had generalised anxiety disorder with a specific pregnancy focus, and it was making her pregnant experience miserable. She was referred to a psychologist who specialised in perinatal mental health. After six sessions of CBT, she described herself as "still cautiously anxious, but no longer consumed by it." She was present at the birth in a way that she told me afterwards she would not have been without treatment. "I was actually there," she said. "I wasn't just terrified."

Your Relationship with Your Own Body

Pregnancy asks something complicated of you in relation to your body: to inhabit it differently, to trust it more deeply, to feel it change in ways over which you have very little control, and to find a way to accommodate those changes with something resembling equanimity.

This is not easy in a culture saturated with images of "post-baby bodies" bouncing back to pre-pregnancy shape within weeks of birth, of celebrities displaying flat stomachs at six weeks postnatal, of an entire industry built around the idea that the changes pregnancy leaves in a woman's body are problems to be corrected rather than evidence of an experience to be honoured.

Let me offer a different frame: your body has done something that no amount of diet or exercise or cosmetic intervention could come close to replicating. It has grown a heart, a brain, a nervous system, a set of kidneys, a pair of lungs, and the most complex organ in biology — the human placenta — from two cells. It has expanded its blood volume by 50%, adapted its cardiovascular system, restructured its immune function, and altered the architecture of its musculoskeletal system — all while you continued to live your ordinary life. And then it has expelled a human being and immediately begun recovering.

The changes this leaves — the stretch marks, the changed shape, the different way your body works — are not flaws. They are records. They tell the story of something extraordinary that your body did.

This is not a call to pretend that body image issues in pregnancy and the postpartum period are not real or do not matter. They are real and they do matter. But if you find yourself spending significant mental energy on the appearance of your postpartum body in ways that are causing distress, that is worth discussing — with your doctor, a counsellor, or someone you trust.

13

Preparing for Baby

The Practical Guide to Getting Ready

Somewhere in the second trimester, the pregnancy transitions from being primarily about you — your body, your symptoms, your feelings — to being also about the person who is coming. You begin to think concretely: Where will the baby sleep? What will I need? Who will help me? How will my life actually change?

This chapter is a practical guide to all of it: the baby's physical environment, the essentials (and non-essentials) of newborn equipment, feeding preparation, and the logistics of the first weeks at home. I want to help you prepare thoughtfully, without succumbing to the anxiety-driven consumerism that the baby industry is extraordinarily good at generating.

The Baby's Sleeping Space

Safe sleeping is the single most important thing to get right for a newborn. The evidence on sudden infant death syndrome (SIDS) is clear on the following points:

The safest sleeping position is on the back. Every time, for every sleep, for the first year. SIDS rates fell by approximately 50% following public health campaigns promoting back sleeping in the 1990s. The concern about choking in the back position is unfounded — healthy babies have airway reflexes that prevent aspiration.

The safest sleeping surface is a firm, flat, clear mattress. No pillows, no loose bedding, no bumpers, no soft toys in the sleeping space. These create suffocation risk.

The safest sleeping environment is the parents' room for the first 6 months. Room-sharing (without bed-sharing) reduces SIDS risk by approximately 50%. The cot or Moses basket should be within arm's reach of your bed.

Bed-sharing has a more complex evidence picture. In Western guidelines it is generally discouraged for the first year, with specific increased risks in the presence of: parents who smoke, parents who have consumed alcohol or sedating medications, premature or low birth weight babies, or very soft sleeping surfaces. In Indian families where bed-sharing is culturally normative and alcohol and smoking are absent, the risks are lower — but the evidence still supports a separate sleeping surface within the parental bed space as the safest arrangement.

Temperature: The room should be 16 to 20°C — perhaps slightly warmer in very cold climates. Overheating is a SIDS risk factor. A useful guide: your baby should be dressed in approximately one more layer than you are comfortable in. Feel the back of the neck or the chest to assess temperature — hands and feet are normally cooler and are not a reliable guide.

What You Actually Need for the Sleeping Space

The baby industry will attempt to sell you a great deal of equipment for your baby's sleeping arrangement. Here is what is actually necessary:

- A firm, flat mattress that fits the cot without gaps at the sides. If using a second-hand cot, buy a new mattress.
- Three to four fitted sheets.
- Two to three cellular blankets or muslin swaddles. Lightweight layers that can be added or removed are safer than heavy blankets.
- A sleeping bag (sleep sack) appropriate to the season and room temperature — rated in togs. These eliminate the risk of loose bedding covering the baby's face.

What you do not need: a pillow (not appropriate for infants under 12 months); a duvet (too warm and too loose); a bumper (suffocation risk); elaborate bedding sets that look beautiful and create hazards.

Feeding Preparation

If You Plan to Breastfeed

Prepare practically: buy two to three well-fitting nursing bras before birth (sized for a cup size larger than your current pregnancy size, as the breasts will be larger when milk comes in). Stock up on breast pads. Purchase a good nipple cream (lanolin-based). Read the breastfeeding chapter of this book (Part 6) before birth, not after — the knowledge will be more accessible when you need it if it is already familiar.

Consider a breastfeeding class before birth — many hospitals and lactation services offer them. Hearing about positioning and latch before your baby arrives means you will have a framework when the actual feeding begins.

Identify a lactation consultant or breastfeeding support service before you need them. Know the name, the phone number, and the hours. Do not wait until day three, when your milk has just come in and you are in pain at 2 a.m., to begin looking for help.

A breast pump: Not everyone needs one immediately, but many women find one valuable in the early weeks — for relieving engorgement, building a supply of expressed milk for when you are away from the baby, or for establishing supply if the baby has difficulty latching. Manual pumps are inexpensive and portable; electric pumps are faster and more effective for regular pumping. Decide which suits your situation and have one available before birth rather than urgently buying one at 4 a.m. on day four.

If You Plan to Formula Feed

Formula feeding is a legitimate and valid choice, and babies fed on formula thrive. If this is your plan, prepare:

- Two to three bottles and teats (newborn-flow teats for newborns)
- Sterilising equipment — a cold-water steriliser, microwave steam steriliser, or electric steriliser

- Choose your formula in advance, but buy only one tin initially — if one brand disagrees with your baby, you will want to switch without having ten tins of an unsuitable formula
- Learn correct preparation: water must be boiled and cooled to no less than 70°C (to kill Cronobacter sakazakii, which can contaminate powdered formula) before adding the powder. Make feeds fresh for each feeding. Discard any unused formula within one hour.

The Newborn Wardrobe: What You Actually Need

The baby clothing industry is a masterclass in generating desire for things that are largely unnecessary. Newborns grow extremely fast — the 0 to 3 month size may be outgrown within 4 to 6 weeks. Here is what is genuinely useful:

- 6 to 8 onesies or jhablas — full-body suits with snap fasteners. The kind that open fully from neck to feet for easy nappy changes at 3 a.m. are worth their weight in gold.
- 3 to 4 sleepsuits or footed onesies for cooler weather
- 4 to 6 pairs of socks (though babies lose these with a commitment and speed that suggests they are doing it on purpose)
- 2 to 3 hats for the hospital and early days (newborns lose heat rapidly through their heads)
- 3 to 4 muslin cloths — for feeding, cleaning up, impromptu sun shading, and dozens of other uses

What you can largely skip: shoes (newborns do not need shoes; their feet need to move freely); formal or decorative outfits (pleasant for photos, impractical for everything else); large quantities of newborn size (many babies arrive too large for newborn clothing and go straight to 0-3 months).

Baby Equipment: The Essential vs the Optional

Truly Essential

- A safe sleeping space — Moses basket, cot, or crib with a firm, new mattress
- Nappies — cloth or disposable. Decide in advance and have a supply. Newborns use 8 to 12 nappies per day. Buy some newborn size and some size 1 — some babies skip newborn size.
- Baby wipes or cotton wool and water (for the newborn period, plain water and cotton wool is gentler on very new skin)
- A changing mat
- A thermometer — a digital ear or underarm thermometer for checking temperature when you are worried
- A car seat if you travel by car — this is non-negotiable for safety and, in many countries, legally required
- A pram or baby carrier — for getting out of the house, which is important for your sanity as well as the baby's

Helpful but Not Essential

- Baby swing or bouncer — some babies are soothed by motion; others are not. Borrow one before buying.
- Baby monitor — if your home is large enough that you cannot hear the baby from another room
- White noise machine — many newborns sleep better with background white noise, mimicking the constant sound environment of the womb. A fan, a white noise app, or a dedicated machine all work.
- Nursing pillow (e.g. a C-shaped pillow) — for positioning the baby comfortably during breastfeeding and bottle feeding

Rarely Worth the Cost

- Wipe warmer — your hands are sufficient

- Expensive nappy bins — an ordinary lidded bin with bags works equally well
- Elaborate baby bath with integrated thermometer — a clean plastic tub and a clean elbow work equally well
- Baby food processor — a fork and a strainer suffice for the first year's purees
- Elaborate nursery decor — your baby does not see well enough in the first months to appreciate the carefully coordinated wallpaper

Preparing Siblings

If you already have a child or children, preparing them for the arrival of a new baby is one of the most important — and most individual — aspects of pregnancy preparation. The response of an existing child to a new sibling depends on age, temperament, the quality of preparation, and the management of the transition.

By Age

Under two years: Children under two have limited capacity to understand the concept of a new sibling in advance. Extensive preparation is less useful and less necessary. Focus on maintaining routine and physical affection after the baby arrives, and minimising unavoidable changes (if you need to move the toddler from a cot to a bed, do it early — not simultaneously with the new baby's arrival).

Two to four years: This age group is typically highly interested in the pregnancy — feeling the bump, "talking to" the baby, going to scans — but has limited capacity to understand long timescales. Tell them about the baby a few months before the due date, not at 12 weeks. Use age-appropriate books about new babies. Involve them in small preparations: choosing a soft toy for the baby, helping fold baby clothes. Prepare them for the fact that newborns are not immediately playmates: "The baby will sleep a lot at first and won't be able to play with you yet, but she will soon."

Five years and older: School-age children can understand much more and can be meaningfully involved. Answer questions honestly at an age-appropriate level. Acknowledge their feelings about the change — including feelings of uncertainty or even resentment, which are completely normal. Give them a specific role: big sister, big brother, baby's protector. Make one-on-one time with each older child a deliberate priority in the postpartum period — even 20 minutes alone with each older child daily protects the relationship significantly.

Whatever the age: tell your existing child about the pregnancy before the physical signs make it obvious, before they hear it from someone else, and before the baby arrives. Children who feel included in the process adjust significantly better than those for whom the baby appears as a fait accompli.

Planning Your Support Network

The single most reliable predictor of a positive postpartum experience — beyond the health of the baby — is the availability of good support. This is not a luxury or a nicety. It is a clinical necessity. Isolated new mothers have significantly higher rates of postpartum depression, breastfeeding failure, and physical complications from inadequate rest.

Before the birth, think concretely about who will help you, in what ways, and for how long:

- Who will stay with you in the first two weeks? Having a family member or trusted friend present to help with cooking, cleaning, and holding the baby while you sleep is invaluable. In Indian families, this is often a grandmother — maternal or paternal — and the traditional practice of the new mother going to her parental home (naiher) for the postnatal period has significant practical wisdom.
- Who is your designated emergency contact outside your partner? If your partner works and you need help during the day, who can you call?

- Who is your paediatrician? Have you chosen one? Have you registered with them? Know their contact number before the baby arrives.
- Who is your postnatal contact for breastfeeding support?
- If you are planning to use paid help — a bai (maid), a nanny, a nighttime nurse or daima — make arrangements well in advance of the due date. Do not leave this to the postpartum period.

✍ My NOTE

I tell every patient at her 32-week appointment: the best thing you can do in the next two months is not buy baby equipment. It is to make a specific, named plan for postnatal support. Who is cooking? Who is cleaning? Who holds the baby at 3 a.m. on the third night? If you cannot answer these questions concretely, the time to solve that problem is now. The baby industry has convinced many women that the preparation for a new baby is primarily about acquiring things. It is not. It is about people.

Birth Plan

A birth plan — or birth preferences, which is the term I prefer, it should express preferences, not demands, and should include a section for "if a caesarean is necessary."

Discussed with your doctor before labour — not presented to a midwife you have never met while you are in active labour.

Labour: Who do you want present? What are your preferences for pain relief — what would you like to try first, what are you open to, what would you prefer to avoid? Do you want to labour in water if available? Are you interested in the birthing ball, TENS machine, or specific positions?

Birth: What are your preferences regarding episiotomy (you can decline if the situation allows, or ask that it be performed only if clinically necessary)? Delayed cord clamping? Who cuts the cord? Immediate skin-to-skin contact?

After delivery: Do you want the baby on your chest immediately? What are your feeding intentions? Are there any medications you want to discuss (e.g. Vitamin K for the baby — recommended; eye drops — depends on local protocol)?

If a caesarean is necessary: Do you want music playing? Do you want the drape lowered so you can see the birth? Immediate skin-to-skin in the operating theatre? Who will be present?

" Reena's Preparation

Reena arrived at her 36-week appointment with a colour-coded folder. Inside: a one-page birth plan, her antenatal records, a printed list of questions, and a note from her mother about the postpartum help she was arranging. I told her it was the most organised preparation I had seen in twenty years of practice. She laughed. "I am a project manager," she said. "I treat everything like a project." Her birth was not, as births rarely are, exactly what the plan described. But her postpartum period was the smoothest I have observed in a first-time mother in a long time — not because of the birth plan, but because of the thought she had given to what she needed and the arrangements she had made to get it. The preparation was the product.

14

Your Questions, My Answers

The Most Common Concerns of Pregnancy

In every pregnancy, there are questions you ask your doctor, questions you are too embarrassed to ask your doctor, questions you ask the internet at midnight (and then regret), and questions you did not know you needed to ask until something unexpected happened. The questions I am asked most frequently across all three trimesters — and answers them honestly, without condescension, and without unnecessary alarm.

No question about your pregnancy is too small, too obvious, or too embarrassing. You are navigating something you have never done before. Questions are the appropriate response.

First Trimester Questions

I had a glass of alcoholic beverages before I knew I was pregnant. Have I harmed my baby?(Specially from high profile, well educated,newly married females from bigger cities)

This is one of the most common and most anxiety-provoking questions I receive, and the honest answer is: almost certainly not. The evidence on alcohol and fetal harm is about sustained, regular drinking — not a single occasion before the pregnancy was known. The embryo, in the very earliest days after fertilisation, follows an "all or nothing" principle: significant alcohol exposure at the moment of fertilisation and before implantation (day 0 to 6) is most likely to result in a failed implantation — the embryo does not survive — rather than a damaged but continuing pregnancy. After implantation but before the neural tube closes (day 14 to 28), the embryo is in the sensitive period for structural development, but again, a single occasion of moderate drinking is not the same as the sustained heavy consumption that causes fetal alcohol spectrum disorder.

The data on occasional alcohol exposure in early unrecognised pregnancy does not show an increased rate of birth defects. This is reassuring. However, because there is no established safe level of alcohol at any point in pregnancy, the recommendation remains: once you know you are pregnant, stop completely. But please do not spend the remainder of your pregnancy in guilt about the glass of wine you had at your friend's wedding at three weeks gestation. The risk is extremely low and the ongoing anxiety is entirely disproportionate to it.

My nausea has suddenly disappeared. Does this mean something is wrong?

The sudden disappearance of nausea is one of the most common triggers of first-trimester panic calls, and it is almost always benign. Here is why it happens: nausea is driven primarily by hCG, which rises steeply from implantation to its peak at around 8 to 10 weeks, and then naturally plateaus and begins to decline. Some women experience this plateau as a sudden improvement in nausea; others notice a more gradual easing. Either is entirely normal. The disappearance of nausea does not mean the pregnancy has ended.

The situation where disappearing nausea genuinely warrants attention is when it is accompanied by other concerning signs: vaginal bleeding, significant cramping, or the disappearance of all pregnancy symptoms simultaneously. In the absence of these, a sudden improvement in nausea around or after 10 weeks is the body's completely normal transition out of the peak hCG phase.

If you are very anxious, it is always reasonable to call your doctor. That is what we are here for. But if your 10-week scan showed a healthy heartbeat and you have now woken up feeling better than you have in two months — enjoy it.

Can I eat street food?

This is a question with enormous cultural weight in India, where street food is a beloved, affordable, and integral part of daily life. The honest answer: street food carries a higher risk of foodborne infection in pregnancy than home-cooked food, and the consequences of certain infections in pregnancy are more severe than they would be outside it. Listeria, salmonella, E. coli — these are not merely inconvenient in pregnancy; they can cause miscarriage, preterm birth, and severe maternal illness.

The risk is not uniform across all street food. The specific concerns are: foods that have been sitting out at room temperature for extended periods (cut fruit, cooked rice and curries kept warm for hours); raw or undercooked elements (runny eggs, raw sprouts, undercooked meat); food prepared with water of uncertain quality; and ice or unboiled water.

Freshly cooked, piping hot street food — food you watch being cooked from fresh ingredients — is significantly safer than pre-prepared food sitting in trays. A freshly made pav bhaji or a just-cooked paratha is a very different proposition from a tray of cut fruit that has been in the sun for three hours. Use judgment. Prioritise freshness. When in doubt, skip it — not because street food is categorically forbidden, but because the risk-benefit calculus in pregnancy has shifted.

I have noticed a brown discharge. Is this a miscarriage?

Brown discharge in early pregnancy is extremely common – it is estimated to affect approximately 20 to 25% of pregnancies in the first trimester. Brown blood is old blood – blood that has taken time to travel from wherever it originated to the vaginal opening, and has oxidised in the process. It is almost always less concerning than fresh bright red bleeding.

The most common cause of first-trimester brown spotting is implantation bleeding – small amounts of blood released as the blastocyst embeds in the uterine wall. Other causes include cervical sensitivity (the cervix has significantly increased blood supply in pregnancy and can bleed with very little provocation – sexual intercourse, a vaginal examination, even a speculum examination), the passage of a small subchorionic haematoma, or simply old blood from early in the pregnancy making its way out.

Brown discharge alone, without cramping and without progression to heavier bright red bleeding, is very unlikely to represent a miscarriage. However, any vaginal bleeding in the first trimester deserves a call to your doctor and an ultrasound assessment to confirm the pregnancy is continuing and to identify the source if possible. Do not dismiss it, but do not catastrophise it either.

Is it safe to travel by air in the first trimester?

Yes. Flying is safe throughout a healthy pregnancy, including the first trimester. The cabin pressure and cosmic radiation exposure of air travel are well within safe limits for pregnant women. The main theoretical concern — radiation exposure — is not a clinically meaningful risk at the levels encountered in ordinary commercial air travel.

Practical considerations for flying in pregnancy: stay well hydrated (aircraft cabins are very dry, and dehydration can trigger Braxton-Hicks contractions in later trimesters); get up and walk the aisle every hour or so to reduce the risk of deep vein thrombosis (DVT), which is elevated in pregnancy; wear compression stockings for long flights; carry your antenatal records and your doctor's contact details.

Individual airlines have varying policies on flying in late pregnancy — most require a letter from your doctor for travel after 28 to 32 weeks and will not allow travel after 36 to 37 weeks without medical clearance. Check with your airline before booking. In the first trimester, no airline restrictions typically apply, and flying is no different in risk than at any other time.

Can I dye my hair in pregnancy?

The evidence on hair dye in pregnancy is reassuring. Studies measuring absorption of hair dye chemicals through the scalp suggest that the amount entering the systemic circulation is very small. No study has demonstrated a clinically meaningful increase in birth defects or pregnancy complications from hair dye use. The chemicals of most concern — aromatic amines — are present in permanent dyes; semi-permanent and temporary dyes use different chemicals with even lower penetration.

The recommendation from most obstetric bodies is: if you want to dye your hair, it is reasonable to wait until after the first trimester (when organogenesis is complete and the embryo is most vulnerable), ensure adequate ventilation during the application, and limit contact time with the scalp. Highlights and balayage techniques, which apply dye away from the scalp, have even lower theoretical risk than full-coverage root-to-tip dye. Henna — natural, without added PPD (p-phenylenediamine) — is considered safe.

I cannot take my iron tablet without vomiting. What should I do?

This is one of the most practically significant medication problems of pregnancy, because iron supplementation is critically important and the tablets are notoriously poorly tolerated. Several approaches can help:

Switch to a different formulation. Ferrous sulphate, the cheapest iron preparation, is also the most likely to cause nausea and constipation. Ferrous bisglycinate (also called iron glycinate) and ferrous gluconate are better tolerated by many women because they release iron more slowly in the gut. These are available at pharmacies and the cost difference is modest. Liquid iron formulations are another option.

Change the timing. Iron tablets cause the most nausea when taken on an empty stomach. If you are taking them first thing in the morning, try taking them after your largest meal of the day instead. The absorption is slightly reduced when taken with food, but a tablet you keep down is better than a tablet you vomit.

Take every other day. Interestingly, a study published in the Lancet in 2017 found that alternate-day iron dosing results in better absorption than daily dosing — because daily iron supplementation upregulates hepcidin, a hormone that blocks iron absorption, whereas skipping a day allows hepcidin levels to fall and the next dose to be absorbed more efficiently.

If you genuinely cannot tolerate oral iron after trying the above: injectable iron (iron sucrose or ferric carboxymaltose) is available and is increasingly used in pregnancy for women who cannot tolerate oral supplementation. A single intravenous iron infusion can correct iron-deficiency anaemia very effectively. Ask your doctor.

Second Trimester Questions

My doctor said my placenta is "low-lying" at the 20-week scan. Should I be worried?

Not yet. A low-lying placenta at 20 weeks is extremely common — found in approximately 2 to 5% of mid-pregnancy scans — and in the vast majority of cases, it resolves without any intervention. Here is why: as the uterus grows throughout the second and third trimesters, its lower segment expands disproportionately more than the upper segment. The placenta, attached to the uterine wall, is carried upward relative to the cervical os (the opening of the cervix) as this expansion occurs. This is called placental migration — though the placenta itself does not move; it is the surrounding tissue that changes.

Studies show that of all placentas described as low-lying or covering the cervical os at 20 weeks, approximately 90 to 95% have completely cleared the os by 32 to 36 weeks. The follow-up scan at 32 to 34 weeks will determine whether this has happened in your case. Only the small minority in whom the placenta still covers the os at this later scan have a diagnosis of placenta praevia requiring specific management (planned caesarean).

In the meantime, if the placenta was described as low-lying or covering the os at 20 weeks, you will typically be advised to avoid penetrative intercourse (to reduce the risk of triggering bleeding), to report any vaginal bleeding promptly, and to attend the follow-up scan as scheduled. These are sensible precautions while awaiting resolution, not evidence that something is seriously wrong.

I keep having vivid and frightening dreams. Is this normal?

Yes, vivid dreams in pregnancy are extremely common — particularly in the first and third trimesters. The causes are multiple: progesterone alters sleep architecture, increasing the proportion of REM sleep (the dreaming phase) and altering its quality; the frequent awakenings of pregnancy (for urination, for discomfort, or for fetal movements) mean that you are more likely to wake during or immediately after a REM period and therefore remember dreams more vividly; and the psychological content of pregnancy — the anxieties, the anticipations, the processing of a major life change — naturally finds expression in dream life.

Vivid, sometimes disturbing dreams about the baby, about labour, about becoming a mother — these are the mind's way of rehearsing, processing, and preparing. They are not omens. They are not predictions. They are not evidence of unconscious hostility toward the pregnancy. They are the dream activity of a person navigating something large and new.

If the dreams are significantly disturbing your sleep or are causing daytime distress, it is worth mentioning to your doctor — particularly if they are accompanied by other symptoms of anxiety. But occasional vivid or alarming dreams, in the context of a healthy pregnancy and an otherwise stable mood, require no treatment beyond the reassurance that they are normal.

My back pain is becoming unmanageable. At what point is this serious?

Back pain in pregnancy is almost universal in some degree, but there are specific red flags that distinguish ordinary musculoskeletal pregnancy back pain from something that requires urgent assessment:

Ordinary pregnancy back pain: Located in the lower back; worse at the end of the day and with prolonged activity; better with rest and position change; no neurological symptoms (no numbness, tingling, or weakness in the legs); no fever; not associated with urinary symptoms.

Back pain requiring urgent assessment: Severe unilateral (one-sided) back pain that radiates down the leg (sciatica or lumbar disc herniation — relatively uncommon but can be severe); back pain associated with fever, urinary symptoms, or burning on urination (possible pyelonephritis — kidney infection); back pain associated with vaginal bleeding or regular contractions (possible placental abruption or preterm labour); acute severe mid-back pain that does not ease with position change (possible pulmonary embolism if right-sided and associated with breathlessness).

For ordinary lower back pain: the evidence-based management is physiotherapy. A physiotherapist trained in pregnancy can assess your specific presentation, provide tailored exercises to strengthen the muscles supporting the spine, and advise on ergonomics, sleeping positions, and activities. A pelvic support belt provides mechanical relief for pelvic girdle pain. Paracetamol is safe. Warm heat packs provide comfort. Swimming offloads the spine beautifully. None of this is a quick fix, but consistent application of these measures significantly reduces the burden of back pain for most women.

I have been told I have gestational diabetes but I feel completely fine. Why do I need to treat it?

Gestational diabetes is, by definition, a condition diagnosed on blood tests in women who feel completely well. The blood glucose elevations it causes are not high enough to produce the classic symptoms of diabetes (extreme thirst, frequent urination, blurred vision) in most women. This is precisely why screening — the 75g OGTT — matters: you cannot identify gestational diabetes from how you feel.

The reason treatment is important despite the absence of symptoms is that the effects of elevated blood glucose in pregnancy operate on the baby, not primarily on the mother. As explained in Part Three of this book: elevated maternal blood glucose crosses the placenta, stimulates fetal insulin production, and causes excessive fetal growth (macrosomia), neonatal hypoglycaemia at birth, and a range of other complications — none of which produce symptoms in the mother. The elevated blood glucose is a problem for your baby even when it causes you no discomfort at all.

Diet management of gestational diabetes is not punitive. It docs not mean starvation or elimination of carbohydrates. It means choosing lower-glycaemic-index carbohydrates (dahl over white rice; roti over maida bread; oats over packaged cereal); distributing carbohydrate intake across three moderate meals and two to three snacks rather than concentrating it in large meals; pairing carbohydrates with protein and fat to slow glucose absorption; and moderating portions of high-glycaemic foods (white rice, white bread, sweet drinks, fruit juice). A dietitian appointment is the most valuable single resource you can access after a GDM diagnosis.

Is it safe to have sex in the second trimester? My husband is worried he will hurt the baby.

The baby cannot be hurt by sexual intercourse. She is in the amniotic sac, surrounded by fluid, separated from the vagina by the thick mucous plug in the cervix. Penetration does not reach the uterus. The uterine contractions triggered by female orgasm are not labour contractions and will not initiate labour in a healthy pregnancy.

The second trimester is, for many couples, the most comfortable trimester for sex — nausea has typically passed, energy has returned, and the bump is not yet large enough to complicate positions significantly. Many women report increased pelvic blood flow and sensitivity in the second trimester that makes sex particularly pleasurable.

The contraindications to sex in pregnancy — placenta praevia, active bleeding, cervical cerclage, ruptured membranes — are specific medical situations that your doctor will inform you of clearly if they apply. In the absence of any of these: sex is safe, and your husband's concern, while sweet, is medically unfounded.

Third Trimester Questions

When should I go to hospital? How do I know if it is real labour?

The general guideline for going to hospital in uncomplicated first labour is the "5-1-1 rule": contractions every 5 minutes, lasting 1 minute, for 1 hour. This combination of frequency, duration, and sustained pattern indicates established active labour rather than irregular early labour or Braxton-Hicks.

For second and subsequent labours, the guideline is more urgent — "3-1-1" (every 3 minutes, lasting 1 minute, for 1 hour), because subsequent labours typically progress faster and can be deceptively advanced when you arrive at hospital.

The signs that should prompt you to go to hospital immediately, regardless of the contraction pattern: vaginal bleeding; your waters breaking (membranes rupturing); significant reduction in fetal movements; a strong gut feeling that something is wrong; and any of the pre-eclampsia warning signs described in Part Seven.

For women who live far from hospital — more than 30 to 45 minutes — err on the side of going earlier. A long journey in active labour is uncomfortable and risky. Know your route, know where to park, know which entrance to use after hours. This knowledge, confirmed before 37 weeks, removes one source of panic from the process.

I am 39 weeks and nothing is happening. What can I do to bring on labour?

This is perhaps the most frequently asked question in late pregnancy, asked with increasing urgency from approximately week 38 onwards. Let me answer it honestly.

The interventions with some evidence: membrane sweeping (also called a stretch and sweep), offered by your doctor from 38 to 39 weeks, involves the doctor inserting a finger through the cervix and making a circular motion to separate the membranes from the lower uterine segment. This releases prostaglandins that can ripen the cervix and initiate labour. It is effective: a Cochrane review found that membrane sweeping reduces the likelihood of formal induction of labour by approximately 50%. It is uncomfortable — sometimes quite significantly — and may cause spotting and irregular contractions for 24 to 48 hours before labour establishes. Ask for it at your 39 or 40-week appointment if it has not already been offered.

Walking: Evidence is mixed, but moderate walking keeps you upright, uses gravity to encourage the baby to descend and press against the cervix, and is definitely not harmful. It is not a powerful labour-initiating intervention, but it is the most recommended practical one.

Sex: Prostaglandins are present in semen, and the mechanical stimulation of the cervix may release prostaglandins locally. The effect is modest, but it is safe, and if you are comfortable and interested, it is reasonable.

The interventions without meaningful evidence: raspberry leaf tea, evening primrose oil, castor oil (this last one can cause diarrhoea and should be avoided — there is no evidence it initiates labour and it makes you feel terrible). Acupuncture and acupressure have low-quality positive evidence from small studies; they are unlikely to harm, and some women find them helpful. Eating dates: a small but genuine evidence base suggests that regular consumption of dates in the last four weeks of pregnancy is associated with higher cervical Bishop scores and spontaneous labour onset. The quantities studied — 6 large dates per day — are achievable.

What is a membrane sweep and does it hurt?

A membrane sweep (stretch and sweep) is a simple procedure performed by your doctor or midwife at an antenatal appointment. A gloved finger is inserted through the cervical os (the opening of the cervix) and moved in a circular motion, sweeping around the lower margin of the uterus to separate the chorioamniotic membranes from the uterine wall. This releases arachidonic acid from the decidua, which is converted to prostaglandins — cervical-ripening agents that can initiate labour.

For the sweep to be performed, the cervix must be accessible — slightly soft, slightly open. A completely closed, posterior, firm cervix cannot be swept; in this case, the doctor may simply attempt cervical assessment and you will be rescheduled.

Does it hurt? This is what most women actually want to know. Honestly: it is uncomfortable, and for some women significantly so. The procedure takes about 30 seconds and the discomfort does not persist beyond that, though cramping and spotting may follow for 24 to 48 hours. Most women describe the sensation as similar to a moderately uncomfortable smear test. A useful framing: a sweep at 39 or 40 weeks is considerably more comfortable than the labour it may help to initiate. If it significantly shortens your time before established labour begins, it is well worth the 30 seconds of discomfort.

After a sweep: wear a pad (spotting is common), expect possible irregular contractions for the rest of the day, and go home and do something distracting. Try not to monitor yourself minutely for the next six hours. If the sweep is going to work, you will know about it. If it is not going to work today, watching carefully will not change that.

My baby is in the breech position at 34 weeks. What are my options?

At 34 weeks, there is still time and opportunity for the baby to turn spontaneously — approximately 70% of breech babies at 32 weeks will have turned to cephalic (head-down) by 36 weeks. Active management of breech position is typically not considered until 36 weeks, when the probability of spontaneous turning has diminished.

At 36 weeks, if the baby remains breech, you will be offered External Cephalic Version (ECV) — a procedure performed in hospital in which a doctor applies firm manual pressure to the outside of your abdomen to rotate the baby head-down. ECV is performed with the benefit of continuous CTG (cardiotocography — fetal heart rate monitoring), under the supervision of a senior obstetrician, with intravenous access in place and the ability to proceed to immediate caesarean if needed. It is not performed at home or in a clinic that cannot manage complications.

ECV success rate: approximately 50 to 65% overall. Factors associated with higher success: non-engagement of the presenting part (the bottom is not yet deep in the pelvis), adequate amniotic fluid, relaxed uterine tone, normal fetal weight, and previous vaginal delivery. Success is lower in first-time mothers, women with anterior placentas, and women with oligohydramnios.

If ECV fails or is declined: planned caesarean section at 38 to 39 weeks is the standard recommendation for uncomplicated breech presentation. Vaginal breech birth is possible in carefully selected cases in centres with specific expertise and experience — it requires an experienced operator, careful fetal position assessment, an adequate pelvis, a normally grown baby, and the woman's fully informed preference. It is not routinely available in most Indian hospitals, and where it is offered, it should be by a team that performs it regularly.

What you can try before 36 weeks to encourage spontaneous turning: hands-and-knees position for 15 to 20 minutes twice daily; swimming; the breech tilt (lying on your back with your hips elevated on pillows); cold applied to the fundal area (where the head is) and warm applied to the lower uterus (to create a temperature gradient the baby may move away from). The evidence for these techniques is limited, but they are harmless, and women often feel better for doing something active. Moxibustion (a traditional Chinese medicine technique involving burning a herb near the acupuncture point BL67 on the little toe) has a small Cochrane review suggesting modest effect; the evidence is weak but the intervention is safe and some women find it worth trying.

I am overdue by five days and my doctor is talking about induction. Is induction safe?

Induction of labour — the artificial initiation of labour using medical interventions — is one of the most extensively studied procedures in obstetrics, and the safety data is reassuring for appropriately timed induction.

The ARRIVE trial, published in 2018, was a landmark study in which 6,000 low-risk women were randomised to either elective induction at 39 weeks or expectant management (waiting for spontaneous labour). The results were counterintuitive: the induction group had a lower caesarean section rate (18.6% vs 22.2%) and no worse neonatal outcomes. This challenged the long-held assumption that induction increases caesarean risk and has influenced obstetric practice globally.

The specific risk of post-term pregnancy (beyond 41 weeks) is stillbirth. Stillbirth rates begin to rise after 40 weeks, and rise more steeply after 42 weeks. The risk at 41 weeks is approximately 1 in 1,000 above the baseline rate; at 42 weeks it is approximately 3 in 1,000 above baseline. These are small absolute numbers, but they represent preventable deaths. The recommendation of most international guidelines — including FOGSI — is to offer induction of labour between 41 and 42 weeks to all women, and to strongly recommend it at 42 weeks.

The method of induction depends on the state of the cervix (Bishop score). An unfavourable cervix (Bishop score below 6) requires cervical ripening first — using prostaglandin gel or pessaries (dinoprostone), misoprostol tablets, or a mechanical balloon catheter. Once the cervix is ripe, oxytocin is given intravenously to establish regular contractions. This process may take 12 to 24 hours from start to established labour, and you should be prepared for the fact that induction is typically not a rapid process.

Contractions from induced labour — particularly with oxytocin — are sometimes described as more intense and less gradual in onset than spontaneous labour contractions. This is because spontaneous labour involves a gradual build of prostaglandins and oxytocin sensitivity, whereas induced labour compresses this build-up. Pain relief should be requested early and without hesitation.

Labour and Birth Questions

What does a contraction actually feel like?

This is the question I am never asked in a consultation but that every first-time mother wants to know. The truthful, unsanitised answer.

Early contractions feel like strong period cramps — the same kind of low central abdominal cramping that many women know from menstruation, but more rhythmic and more consistent. They come in waves: building to a peak over 20 to 30 seconds, holding for a few seconds, then releasing. Between them, you feel entirely normal.

Active labour contractions are different in character as well as intensity. They are longer (60 to 90 seconds), stronger, and more consuming. Many women feel them in the back as well as the abdomen — a tightening that wraps around, starting in the lower back and gripping across the front. At the peak, they require your full attention. You cannot speak through them. You can breathe through them, and this breathing is the most useful thing you will do in labour.

The sensations that are hardest to convey: the pressure — an enormous, downward, expulsive pressure, particularly in the transition phase and second stage, that is unlike any other physical sensation. The burning, stretching sensation of crowning — the so-called "ring of fire" — that most women describe as intense but manageable because it is so clearly associated with progress, with the baby arriving. The extraordinary relief of the baby's body emerging after the head — the sudden end of the downward pressure, replaced by an extraordinary feeling of completeness.

What I want you to know: contractions are painful, but the pain is not the same as injury pain. It is purposeful pain — your uterus working, your cervix opening, your baby descending. Many women find that understanding this — knowing that each contraction is progress, that each wave of intensity is finite, that the body is doing exactly what it is designed to do — changes the quality of the experience. You are not a passive victim of the pain. You are working. That distinction matters.

Can I eat and drink during labour?

Guidelines on eating and drinking in labour have evolved significantly in the last two decades. The traditional restriction — nothing by mouth from early labour — was based on Mendelson's syndrome: aspiration of gastric contents into the lungs during general anaesthesia, a serious complication of obstetric anaesthesia in the mid-20th century when general anaesthesia for caesarean was much more common and anaesthetic techniques were less sophisticated.

With modern anaesthetic practice — rapid sequence induction, much more widespread use of regional (spinal/epidural) rather than general anaesthesia for caesarean, and improved airway management techniques — the risk of Mendelson's syndrome is dramatically lower. And the evidence on food and fluid restriction in labour is clear: it does not improve maternal outcomes, and it imposes real costs — hunger and thirst increase anxiety and pain perception, reduce stamina, and may deplete the energy reserves needed for prolonged labour and the pushing stage.

Current RCOG and ACOG guidelines support free clear fluid intake throughout labour for low-risk women. The FOGSI position is similar. Many hospitals restrict solid food during active labour as a precaution against the (small but non-zero) chance of emergency caesarean under general anaesthesia — eating light, easily digestible food in early labour is generally supported, with progressively more caution as labour advances.

Practically: eat something in early labour before you come to hospital (toast, banana, yoghurt, plain rice). Drink regularly throughout — water, diluted juice, coconut water, ice chips. If your hospital restricts solid food once admitted, this is a reasonable policy; stay hydrated regardless.

I am terrified of tearing. What can I do to reduce the risk?

Fear of perineal tearing is one of the most common specific fears about birth, and it is not irrational — perineal trauma affects a significant proportion of women who deliver vaginally. But there are interventions that genuinely reduce both the risk and severity of tearing, and understanding them gives you practical agency.

Perineal massage: Performed from 35 weeks for 5 to 10 minutes daily, perineal massage involves using clean, lubricated fingers (you, your partner, or oil — olive, almond, coconut) to stretch the perineal tissue, progressively increasing the stretch over weeks. The technique involves pressing downward toward the rectum, holding the stretch for 1 to 2 minutes, then slowly moving side to side. The evidence: a Cochrane review found that perineal massage from 35 weeks reduces the risk of third and fourth degree tears in first-time mothers by approximately 10%, and significantly reduces the risk of episiotomy. These are meaningful effects, and the investment is 5 minutes a day.

Warm compress in second stage: Application of a warm compress to the perineum by the midwife or doctor during the pushing phase reduces the risk of severe perineal trauma. The heat promotes tissue elasticity and reduces the inflammatory response to stretching. Midwives trained in physiological birth use this routinely.

Controlled delivery of the head: A slow, controlled delivery of the baby's head — guided by the midwife or doctor asking you to pant rather than push at crowning, to allow the perineum to stretch gradually — significantly reduces the risk of severe tears compared with an uncontrolled, rapid delivery. Panting at crowning is counterintuitive when every instinct is screaming to push — but it works.

Upright or kneeling positions: Delivering in an upright, forward-leaning, or kneeling position (rather than lithotomy — lying on your back with legs raised) has been consistently associated with lower rates of severe perineal trauma in multiple studies. The biomechanics make sense: upright positions align the baby's descent with the natural curve of the pelvis, and the perineum is under less tension than in the supine position.

Episiotomy: Routine episiotomy — cutting the perineum to widen the opening — has been clearly shown in multiple randomised controlled trials to not protect against severe tears and to cause more harm than selective episiotomy. It is not protective. A selective episiotomy — performed specifically when the baby needs to be delivered quickly or when a severe tear appears unavoidable — remains appropriate, but the routine use of episiotomy in normal birth is not supported by evidence and should be questioned.

15

Your Tests and Investigations Explained

Every Test, What It Measures, and Why It Matters

Pregnancy involves a remarkable number of blood tests, scans, swabs, and monitoring procedures — many of which are offered with minimal explanation. This chapter explains every standard test of the antenatal period: what is being measured, what the results mean, what happens if the result is abnormal, and why each test matters to your health and your baby's.

Understanding your tests transforms you from a passive recipient of results into an informed participant in your care. When you understand why a test is being done and what a normal result looks like, an abnormal result is less frightening — because you know what it means and what the next step is.

Blood Tests

Full Blood Count (FBC / CBC)

The full blood count is performed at the booking visit, at 28 weeks, and sometimes at 36 weeks. It measures three cell populations in the blood:

Haemoglobin (Hb) — the iron-containing protein in red blood cells that carries oxygen. The WHO defines anaemia in pregnancy as haemoglobin below 11 g/dL in the first and third trimesters and below 10.5 g/dL in the second trimester (due to physiological haemodilution). FOGSI recommends targeting a haemoglobin above 11 g/dL throughout pregnancy. A haemoglobin below 8 g/dL is severe anaemia and requires urgent treatment.

Mean Corpuscular Volume (MCV) — the average size of red blood cells. In iron-deficiency anaemia, red cells are small (microcytic) and the MCV is low (below 80 fL). In folate or Vitamin B12 deficiency, red cells are large (macrocytic) and the MCV is high (above 100 fL). A normal MCV in an anaemic woman suggests either early iron deficiency (before the cells have had time to become small), mixed deficiency (iron plus folate), or a non-nutritional cause.

White blood cell count (WBC) — the infection-fighting cells. A modest rise in white cells during pregnancy is normal (the normal range in pregnancy is higher than in non-pregnant adults). A very high or rapidly rising WBC, particularly if accompanied by fever and clinical signs, suggests infection.

Platelets — cells involved in blood clotting. Gestational thrombocytopenia — a mild fall in platelets that occurs in approximately 5 to 8% of pregnancies — is a benign condition that does not require treatment and does not affect labour or delivery. Significant thrombocytopenia (platelets below 100 x 10^9/L) requires investigation for underlying causes (immune thrombocytopenia, HELLP syndrome, antiphospholipid syndrome) and specialist input.

Blood Group and Antibody Screen

Your ABO blood group (A, B, AB, or O) and Rh (D) status are determined at the booking visit. The Rh (D) status — positive or negative — is particularly important.

Approximately 15% of Indian women are Rh negative. If you are Rh negative and your baby is Rh positive — which can happen if your partner carries the Rh positive gene — small amounts of fetal blood can enter your circulation at delivery (or at other sensitising events: miscarriage, ectopic pregnancy, antepartum haemorrhage, amniocentesis, ECV). Your immune system, encountering the Rh positive antigen for the first time, may develop anti-D antibodies.

In the current pregnancy, first-time sensitisation rarely causes problems because the antibody response develops too slowly. But in a subsequent Rh positive pregnancy, the already-primed immune system produces a rapid, high-level antibody response. These antibodies cross the placenta and destroy the baby's Rh positive red blood cells — causing haemolytic disease of the fetus and newborn (HDFN), which can range from mild jaundice to severe anaemia, heart failure, and fetal death.

Prevention: Anti-D immunoglobulin injection, given at 28 weeks and again at 34 weeks (prophylactically) and within 72 hours of any potentially sensitising event, neutralises any fetal Rh positive cells in the maternal circulation before the immune system can mount a response. It is a simple, safe, and highly effective intervention that has virtually eliminated HDFN in the countries where it is systematically applied. If you are Rh negative, these injections are not optional.

The antibody screen — also performed at booking and at 28 weeks — tests the blood for any alloantibodies (immune antibodies against blood group antigens). The most important is anti-D (as above), but other antibodies (anti-c, anti-Kell, anti-E) can cause similar problems and are equally screened for.

Thyroid Function (TSH, Free T4)

TSH — thyroid-stimulating hormone — is the pituitary hormone that controls thyroid activity. It is the most sensitive indicator of thyroid function: a high TSH means the pituitary is working hard to drive an underactive thyroid (hypothyroidism); a low TSH means the pituitary is suppressing an overactive thyroid (hyperthyroidism).

Hypothyroidism in pregnancy: The target TSH in pregnancy is lower than outside of pregnancy — below 2.5 mIU/L in the first trimester, below 3.0 mIU/L in the second and third. Above these levels, thyroid function is considered suboptimal and treatment with levothyroxine is generally recommended. The reason for the lower threshold in pregnancy: the fetus depends entirely on maternal thyroid hormone transfer in the first trimester (the fetal thyroid does not become functional until 10 to 12 weeks), and adequate thyroid hormone is essential for fetal brain development.

Hyperthyroidism in pregnancy: A low TSH in pregnancy requires careful interpretation. TSH is physiologically suppressed in normal early pregnancy because hCG (which is structurally similar to TSH) cross-reacts with the TSH receptor and mildly stimulates the thyroid — this is "gestational hyperthyroidism" and is normal, requiring no treatment. True hyperthyroidism (Graves' disease) produces a suppressed TSH alongside elevated free T4 and T3, and requires treatment. Untreated hyperthyroidism is associated with preterm birth, fetal growth restriction, and neonatal thyroid problems.

Women with pre-existing thyroid disease on thyroid medication before pregnancy should have their TSH checked at the first antenatal appointment and every 4 weeks for the first half of pregnancy — because thyroid requirements typically increase in pregnancy and the dose of levothyroxine almost always needs to be increased.

Blood Glucose and HbA1c

The booking glucose test — whether a fasting glucose, random glucose, or HbA1c — screens for pre-existing, undiagnosed type 2 diabetes or pre-diabetes. As discussed extensively in the nutrition and complications chapters, undiagnosed diabetes in early pregnancy is associated with a significantly elevated risk of congenital malformations (because the embryo is developing in a high-glucose environment during the critical organogenesis period).

HbA1c (glycated haemoglobin) reflects average blood glucose over the preceding 2 to 3 months. An HbA1c above 48 mmol/mol (6.5%) indicates diabetes; between 39 and 47 mmol/mol (5.7% to 6.4%) indicates pre-diabetes. In pregnancy, HbA1c is interpreted with care — the physiological haemodilution and increased red cell turnover of pregnancy can lower HbA1c independently of glucose levels.

The 75g OGTT at 24 to 28 weeks is the standard screening test for gestational diabetes (which by definition develops in pregnancy and is not present before). The diagnostic criteria and management are covered in detail in Part Three.

Vitamin D Level

A 25-hydroxyvitamin D (25-OH-D) level below 50 nmol/L (20 ng/mL) indicates insufficiency; below 25 nmol/L (10 ng/mL) indicates deficiency. The target in pregnancy is above 50 nmol/L, ideally above 75 nmol/L (30 ng/mL).

As discussed in Part Eight, Vitamin D deficiency is extraordinarily prevalent in India — 70 to 90% of women in many studies — and carries genuine pregnancy risks. The routine measurement of Vitamin D level at the booking visit is increasingly recommended in Indian practice, because the dose of supplementation required to achieve adequate levels varies widely: a woman with a level of 45 nmol/L needs a different supplementation strategy than one with a level of 8 nmol/L.

The currently available Vitamin D supplements in India include cholecalciferol (D3) — the preferred form — in doses of 1,000, 2,000, 60,000 IU (a common high-dose oral sachet), and 600,000 IU injectable ampules. For mild insufficiency (25 to 50 nmol/L), daily supplementation with 1,000 to 2,000 IU is appropriate. For significant deficiency (below 25 nmol/L), a higher loading regimen under medical supervision is more appropriate.

Iron Studies

A full blood count tells you the haemoglobin level — the end result of iron status — but iron studies give you the earlier picture, identifying iron depletion before anaemia has developed. The key parameters:

Serum ferritin — the iron storage protein. It reflects iron stores. A ferritin below 30 ng/mL indicates iron store depletion, even in the absence of anaemia. A ferritin below 12 ng/mL indicates iron deficiency. In pregnancy, a ferritin below 30 ng/mL warrants iron supplementation even if haemoglobin is normal — because iron stores are depleted and, without supplementation, anaemia will develop as pregnancy progresses.

Ferritin can be falsely elevated in inflammatory conditions (it is an acute phase protein); a C-reactive protein (CRP) measurement alongside ferritin helps interpretation.

Serum iron and Transferrin Saturation — measure the circulating iron and its binding to transferrin (the transport protein). These are more variable across the day and less reliable than ferritin as markers of iron status. They are mainly used in conjunction with ferritin to confirm iron deficiency when clinical decisions about IV iron are being made.

Reticulocyte haemoglobin content (CHr or Ret-He) — measured on modern automated blood counters — reflects the iron available for haemoglobin synthesis in newly produced red cells and is an early, sensitive marker of iron-restricted erythropoiesis. It is increasingly used to guide decisions about iron supplementation during pregnancy.

Urine Tests

Urine Culture (MSU)

The midstream urine (MSU) culture at the booking visit screens for asymptomatic bacteriuria (ASB) — the presence of bacteria in the urine at significant counts ($\geq 10^5$ colony-forming units/mL) in the absence of any symptoms. It affects 2 to 7% of pregnant women.

Left untreated, ASB in pregnancy progresses to symptomatic UTI in approximately 30% of cases and to pyelonephritis (kidney infection) in 20 to 25%. Pyelonephritis is associated with a significantly elevated risk of preterm labour, maternal sepsis, and in severe cases, adult respiratory distress syndrome. Treating ASB with a 3 to 7 day course of appropriate antibiotics (guided by sensitivity testing) reduces the risk of pyelonephritis by over 90%.

This is one of the clearest examples of a screening test whose benefit is so substantial that it should be universal in pregnancy.

A urine culture costs a few hundred rupees. Treating pyelonephritis costs vastly more, in money, in hospital time, and in risk.

Urine dipstick for protein: Tested at every antenatal appointment, because protein in the urine (proteinuria) is one of the hallmarks of pre-eclampsia. A trace of protein on dipstick is often a laboratory or collection artefact; significant proteinuria (1+ or more) warrants a formal measurement by protein/creatinine ratio or 24-hour urine collection, alongside blood pressure measurement.

Urine dipstick for glucose: Glucose in the urine (glycosuria) in pregnancy may simply reflect the lower renal threshold for glucose reabsorption described earlier — this is physiological and does not diagnose gestational diabetes. However, persistent glycosuria — particularly on multiple occasions — warrants formal glucose testing if the OGTT has not already been performed.

Ultrasound Scans

The Dating Scan (7–10 Weeks)

The first-trimester dating scan confirms the pregnancy is in the uterus (not ectopic), identifies the heartbeat, measures the crown-rump length (CRL) to establish gestational age, and checks for multiple pregnancy. If the CRL-based date differs from the LMP date by more than 5 days, the scan date is used for all subsequent calculations — ensuring consistent dating throughout pregnancy.

Expected findings at 7 to 10 weeks: a single gestational sac with a yolk sac, a visible fetal pole with a flickering heartbeat, and a CRL corresponding to the gestational age. A heartbeat rate below 100 beats per minute at this stage is associated with an increased risk of miscarriage and warrants close follow-up. The absence of a heartbeat when the CRL is above 7 mm confirms a missed miscarriage.

Subchorionic haematoma — blood pooling between the chorion and the uterine wall — is seen as a dark, crescent-shaped area adjacent to the gestational sac. Its clinical significance depends on its size relative to the gestational sac: a small haematoma (less than a third of the sac circumference) carries little increased risk; a large haematoma (more than two-thirds) is associated with an elevated miscarriage risk. Most small haematomas resolve spontaneously.

The NT Scan (11+0 to 13+6 Weeks)

The nuchal translucency scan is covered in detail in Part Two. Additional structures assessed at this scan that are worth knowing:

Nasal bone: Absent or hypoplastic nasal bone is present in approximately 60 to 70% of Down syndrome fetuses (compared with about 2% of chromosomally normal fetuses). Its assessment improves the sensitivity of combined first-trimester screening by approximately 5 to 10%.

Tricuspid regurgitation: Tricuspid regurgitation — backflow through the tricuspid valve of the fetal heart — is found in approximately 65% of Down syndrome fetuses at this gestational age, compared with 1 to 2% of normal fetuses. Its assessment requires specific equipment and training and is not performed at all centres.

Ductus venosus flow: Abnormal ductus venosus flow (reversed A-wave) at 11 to 14 weeks is associated with chromosomal abnormalities and major cardiac defects. Combined with NT and nasal bone, it significantly increases the sensitivity of first-trimester screening.

Crown-rump length (for dating): Measured at this scan to confirm or refine gestational age. The NT measurement is only valid when the CRL is between 45 and 84 mm — the specific window corresponds to the gestational age window of 11+0 to 13+6 weeks.

The 20-Week Anomaly Scan

The anomaly scan is covered extensively in Part Three. One additional aspect worth discussing: incidental maternal findings. The anomaly scan occasionally identifies findings in the mother as well as the baby — ovarian cysts, uterine fibroids, or pelvic masses — that were not the purpose of the examination but require follow-up. These findings are not rare; large fibroids are present in approximately 5 to 10% of pregnancies and are often first identified at the anomaly scan. Your doctor will explain any such findings and advise on their clinical significance.

Growth Scans (28–36 Weeks)

Third-trimester growth scans measure the following parameters to estimate fetal weight and assess wellbeing:

Biparietal diameter (BPD): The width of the fetal head at its widest point, measured transversely across the skull. One of the four standard biometric measurements.

Head circumference (HC): A more reliable measurement of head size than BPD alone, as it is less affected by the shape of the head (which varies between fetuses).

Abdominal circumference (AC): The circumference of the fetal abdomen at the level of the liver, measured in cross-section. This is the most clinically significant biometric measurement for fetal growth assessment — it reflects liver size (and therefore glycogen stores) and subcutaneous fat, both of which are affected early in fetal growth restriction and in macrosomia.

Femur length (FL): The length of the fetal femur (thigh bone). Used as a proxy for overall fetal long bone growth.

These four measurements are entered into an algorithm that calculates the estimated fetal weight (EFW). The EFW is compared to gestational-age-specific reference charts and plotted as a centile — the 10th centile baby is larger than 10% of babies and smaller than 90% at that gestational age. A baby below the 10th centile is small for gestational age (SGA); above the 90th centile is large for gestational age (LGA).

It is important to understand that centile at a single measurement is less clinically meaningful than the trajectory of growth over time. A baby consistently on the 8th centile but growing at a normal rate (following the centile line) is likely a constitutionally small but healthy baby. A baby who was on the 45th centile at 28 weeks but has fallen to the 12th centile at 34 weeks has crossed centile lines downward — this is fetal growth restriction until proven otherwise, and requires Doppler assessment and increased monitoring.

Cervical and Vaginal Tests

Group B Streptococcus (GBS) Swab

Group B Streptococcus (Streptococcus agalactiae, GBS) is a bacterium that colonises the rectum and vagina of approximately 10 to 30% of women asymptomatically. The woman herself is entirely unaffected. But GBS can be transmitted to the baby during labour and delivery, causing early-onset neonatal GBS disease — a serious infection that can cause neonatal sepsis, pneumonia, and meningitis, and is associated with significant morbidity and mortality.

Two strategies exist for preventing early-onset GBS disease:

Universal screening (risk-based in India, more widely offered in higher-income settings): A combined low vaginal and anorectal swab is taken at 35 to 37 weeks and cultured for GBS. Women who test positive are offered intravenous benzylpenicillin in labour — given from the onset of labour or 4 hours before delivery, it dramatically reduces the risk of GBS transmission to the baby. Women who test negative do not need intrapartum antibiotics.

Risk-factor-based approach (used in the UK and many Indian centres): Intrapartum antibiotics are given to women with specific risk factors — preterm labour, prolonged rupture of membranes (more than 18 hours), maternal fever in labour, or GBS bacteriuria in the current pregnancy — without universal screening. This approach identifies fewer at-risk women than universal screening but avoids the cost and unnecessary antibiotic exposure of screening all women.

Ask your doctor or hospital which approach they use and whether a GBS swab will be offered.

Cervical Length Measurement

Transvaginal cervical length measurement — using a vaginal ultrasound probe to measure the length of the cervix from internal os to external os — is the most accurate predictor of preterm birth risk available. A short cervix (below 25 mm) between 18 and 24 weeks identifies women at significantly elevated risk of preterm birth.

Cervical length measurement is recommended for women with a previous preterm birth (below 34 weeks), previous mid-trimester loss (second-trimester miscarriage), or uterine anomalies. Some units offer it universally at the 20-week scan; this is evidence-based and valuable when practical.

A cervical length below 25 mm at 18 to 24 weeks in a singleton pregnancy qualifies for vaginal progesterone supplementation, which has been shown in high-quality trials to reduce preterm birth before 33 weeks by approximately 45%.

Fetal Monitoring

CTG — Cardiotocography

The CTG is the electronic fetal heart rate monitor — the machine with two sensors attached to the abdomen that produces the continuous paper printout of fetal heart rate and uterine contractions. It is the primary method of fetal surveillance in labour and in antenatal assessments of fetal wellbeing.

The CTG displays two traces: the upper trace (fetal heart rate) and the lower trace (uterine contractions). A normal fetal heart rate trace has the following features:

Baseline rate: 110 to 160 beats per minute. A rate below 110 (bradycardia) or above 160 (tachycardia) requires assessment of cause and possibly intervention.

Baseline variability: The normal "wiggly" nature of the trace — the normal heart rate fluctuates by 5 to 25 beats per minute around the baseline. This variability reflects the normal autonomic nervous system tone of a well-oxygenated fetus. Reduced variability (below 5 bpm for more than 50 minutes) is concerning and warrants urgent assessment.

Accelerations: Brief rises in the fetal heart rate of at least 15 beats per minute above the baseline, lasting at least 15 seconds. The presence of at least two accelerations in 20 minutes is a reassuring sign of fetal wellbeing. Their absence (non-reactive trace) requires further assessment.

Decelerations: Falls in the fetal heart rate below the baseline. Early decelerations (falling with contractions and recovering before the contraction ends) are benign — caused by vagal stimulation from head compression. Variable decelerations are caused by umbilical cord compression. Late decelerations (beginning after the contraction peak and recovering after the contraction ends) are the most concerning pattern — they are associated with uteroplacental insufficiency and fetal hypoxia when persistent.

Interpretation of CTG is a skill that requires training and experience. Do not attempt to interpret your own CTG trace from the printout. If your doctor or midwife expresses concern about the trace, trust their assessment and ask them to explain what they are seeing. The language of CTG is clear and specific, and there is no reason you cannot understand the explanation.

Biophysical Profile (BPP)

The biophysical profile is an ultrasound-based assessment of fetal wellbeing, typically performed when CTG or Doppler findings raise concern about fetal status. It assesses five parameters, each scored 0 or 2:

- Fetal breathing movements — at least one episode of 30 seconds or more in 30 minutes
- Fetal movements — at least 3 body or limb movements in 30 minutes
- Fetal tone — at least one episode of extension with return to flexion
- Amniotic fluid volume — at least one pocket of fluid measuring 2 cm or more
- Non-reactive CTG — scored as 0 if a reactive CTG is included in the BPP

A score of 8 to 10 is reassuring. A score of 6 may warrant repeat in 6 hours. A score of 4 or below, particularly if fluid is reduced, is associated with significant fetal compromise and usually prompts delivery.

The BPP reflects the fetal response to hypoxia: the breathing centre in the brain is the most sensitive to oxygen deprivation and is the first to become inactive (disappearance of breathing movements), followed by the movement and tone centres. Amniotic fluid volume is a long-term indicator of fetal renal function — persistent oligohydramnios suggests chronic placental insufficiency. The hierarchical scoring of the BPP therefore reflects the severity and chronicity of any fetal compromise.

✍ My NOTE

I am sometimes asked: "How do I know my baby is okay in between my appointments?" The answer is fetal movements. A healthy, well-oxygenated baby at 28 weeks and beyond moves every day, with a pattern that is individual to that baby. You know your baby's normal activity level better than I do. If it changes — if the movements seem less frequent, less vigorous, or qualitatively different — that is the signal to call. Not to wait until tomorrow. Not to drink cold water and wait. To call. The stories that stay with me in obstetrics are not the ones where women came in unnecessarily. They are the ones where they waited too long.

The First Hour After Birth

The Golden Hour,The room changes before you do.

One moment there is noise , instructions, instruments, pressure, movement, people speaking quickly around you — and then suddenly, there is a cry. Sharp, wet, startled, indignant. A sound unlike any other sound you have ever heard, because your body recognises it before your mind does.

Your baby is here.

For months, this child existed in shadows and abstractions: scan images, kicks beneath your ribs, names discussed in whispers at night. And now suddenly there is a real human being in the room warm, slippery, breathing, crying, alive.

Many women expect the dominant emotion at birth to be immediate overwhelming joy. Sometimes it is. Sometimes it is relief. Sometimes disbelief. Sometimes exhaustion so profound that emotion arrives several minutes later, quietly and all at once. Some women cry immediately. Some stare silently. Some laugh. Some ask practical questions. Some simply close their eyes because they have nothing left in them for a few moments except survival. All of these reactions are normal. Birth is not a performance. There is no correct emotional script.

The First Minute of Life

The moment after birth represents one of the most dramatic physiological transitions in human existence. Until seconds ago, your baby was living in an aquatic environment entirely dependent on the placenta for oxygen, temperature regulation, and nutrition. The lungs were filled with fluid. Blood bypassed them through specialised fetal circulation pathways — the ductus arteriosus and foramen ovale. Then the umbilical cord is clamped. And everything changes. The first breath your baby takes is extraordinarily hard work. The lungs must expand for the first time against resistance, clearing fluid from millions of tiny alveoli. Oxygen levels rise rapidly. Blood vessels inside the lungs open. Fetal circulation begins shutting down and newborn circulation begins. That first cry is not merely emotional. It is physiological survival.

♥ YOUR BABY RIGHT NOW Minutes old

Your baby's skin may appear bluish initially around the hands and feet , this is called acrocyanosis and is normal in the first hours of life. The head may look elongated or swollen after vaginal delivery due to molding of the skull bones during passage through the birth canal. There may be vernix ,a white creamy protective coating, still present in skin folds. The eyes may be swollen. Female babies may have enlarged labia from maternal hormones; male babies may have swollen scrotums. None of this means anything is wrong. Newborns are not polished creatures. They are freshly born mammals adapting to air, light, gravity, sound, and touch for the first time.

Skin-to-Skin: Why It Matters So Much

If both mother and baby are stable, your baby should be placed directly on your chest immediately after birth — skin against skin, covered together with a warm blanket.

This practice, once considered optional, is now recognised as one of the most biologically important interventions in newborn care.

Skin-to-skin contact:

stabilises the baby's temperature, regulates heart rate and breathing,reduces crying, lowers maternal stress hormones, improves blood glucose stability, increases breastfeeding success, and strengthens maternal-infant bonding.

Your chest is not simply a place to hold the baby. Physiologically, it functions almost like an external womb in the first hour after birth.

Remarkably, studies show a mother's chest temperature can actually rise or fall by 1–2°C in response to the baby's temperature needs. Your body has already begun mothering before you consciously know how.

✍ My NOTE.

One of the most beautiful things I have ever watched in medicine is the instinctive behaviour of a healthy newborn placed skin-to-skin after birth. If left undisturbed, many babies will slowly crawl toward the breast, bobbing their heads, opening their mouths, searching blindly for milk they have never tasted before. No one teaches them this. Biology does.

The Placenta The Organ You Grew and Will Never See Again

After your baby is born, the uterus continues contracting. Within a few minutes, these contractions separate the placenta from the uterine wall.

You may feel: cramping, pressure, or a brief urge to push again.

Delivery of the placenta is usually quick and far less painful than delivery of the baby. And yet medically, this stage matters enormously. The placenta is an extraordinary temporary organ. grown entirely for this pregnancy and discarded afterwards. It acted simultaneously as: lung, kidney, liver, immune interface, hormone factory, and nutritional support system. For months, it kept two circulatory systems alive without allowing their blood to directly mix. Few biological systems in medicine are more sophisticated. After delivery, your doctor examines the placenta carefully to ensure it is complete. Retained placental fragments can cause severe postpartum bleeding and infection.

The Uterus After Delivery Immediately after birth, your uterus contracts powerfully to compress the blood vessels that supplied the placenta during pregnancy.

This contraction is critical. During pregnancy, approximately 500–750 mL of blood per minute flowed through the uterus.

Once the placenta detaches, those vessels are suddenly exposed. Without strong uterine contraction, dangerous hemorrhage can occur rapidly.

This is why your abdomen may be firmly massaged after delivery. It can feel uncomfortable, but it helps the uterus remain contracted.

Oxytocin either naturally released or given as an injection plays a major role here. Oxytocin is often called the "love hormone," but physiologically it is also the "survival hormone" of childbirth:

it contracts the uterus, reduces bleeding, stimulates milk let-down, and enhances emotional bonding. The same hormone helping you fall in love with your baby is also preventing hemorrhage.

THE SCIENCE BEHIND IT

Why Mothers Shake After Delivery

Many women begin shaking uncontrollably after birth, even when they are not cold. This is extremely common.

Postpartum shaking occurs because: adrenaline levels fall suddenly after labour,the nervous system is discharging stress hormones,blood vessels are rapidly changing tone, fluid shifts are occurring, and body temperature regulation is adjusting after intense exertion.

The shaking may look dramatic but is usually harmless and resolves within minutes to hours.

What You Might Be Feeling

Immediately after birth, you may experience: intense relief,

emotional numbness, trembling, thirst, exhaustion, overwhelming protectiveness, disbelief that the baby is finally outside your body, sudden fear about responsibility,

or an unexpected calmness. Many mothers repeatedly check whether the baby is breathing. This is normal.

Your brain is adapting rapidly to maternal vigilance a deeply biological protective mechanism.

The First Breastfeed

The first milk your breasts produce is called colostrum.

It is: thick, yellow-golden, concentrated, and produced in very small quantities.This is normal.

A newborn stomach on day one is tiny approximately the size of a cherry. Large milk volumes are neither expected nor needed initially. Colostrum is extraordinarily rich in: antibodies (especially IgA), immune cells, growth factors, protein, and protective molecules lining the newborn intestine.

It is often called "liquid gold," and scientifically the description is justified. The first feed may happen easily. Or it may not.

Some babies latch immediately. Some are sleepy. Some struggle. Some mothers feel confident instantly. Some feel awkward and frightened. All of this is normal. Breastfeeding is natural, but it is also learned.

" Meera's First Hour

"I thought I would instantly know how to hold him," Meera told me later. "Instead I looked at the nurse and said, 'Please don't let me drop him.'"

She had laboured for fourteen hours. Her hair was stuck to her face with sweat. She looked completely exhausted.

And then the baby opened his eyes while lying on her chest.

"That was the moment," she said quietly. "Not the delivery. Not the crying. That. When he looked at me."

The First Night as Parents

Hospitals are strange places at night.

Corridors quieten but never become silent. Somewhere, a monitor continues beeping. A newborn cries two rooms away. Nurses walk softly under dimmed lights. The world outside has gone to sleep, but inside the maternity ward, entirely new lives are beginning. And in one of those beds, usually exhausted beyond language, are two people staring at a baby and thinking the same stunned thought:

"They are letting us take care of this child ourselves."

The first night after birth has a peculiar emotional atmosphere. Time behaves differently. You may feel as though labour happened years ago and ten minutes ago simultaneously. Your body is sore, swollen, trembling with fatigue. Your mind is overstimulated. Your emotions are fluctuating rapidly between awe and fear and tenderness and complete disbelief.

And beside you — in a plastic bassinet or sleeping against your chest — is the person who has reorganised your entire life in a single day.

♥ YOUR BABY RIGHT NOW 6–24 hours old.

Your baby is adapting continuously to life outside the uterus. The lungs are clearing residual fluid. Blood circulation is shifting permanently into newborn patterns. Blood sugar regulation, temperature control, feeding reflexes, and sleep cycles are all stabilising for the first time.

Newborns in the first 24 hours are often surprisingly alert immediately after birth, followed by long periods of sleepiness. This is normal. Birth is physiologically exhausting for babies too.

You may notice: irregular breathing, brief pauses under 10 seconds, sneezing, hiccups, stretching, startling movements, or noisy breathing. Most of these are normal newborn adjustment behaviours.

The Strange Silence After Labour

Many women describe an unexpected emotional emptiness after delivery, not sadness exactly, but a strange quietness. For months, pregnancy filled every hour: kicks, scans, anticipation, discomfort, counting weeks, planning labour, imagining birth. And suddenly the central event is over. The baby is outside. The waiting has ended.

Your body and brain now begin an abrupt transition from "pregnant" to "postpartum," and hormonally this is one of the most dramatic endocrine shifts in human physiology.

Within hours after delivery: progesterone levels fall sharply, estrogen levels collapse, oxytocin surges, prolactin rises, cortisol fluctuates, adrenaline dissipates. The emotional consequences of this hormonal transition are enormous.

This is why many mothers cry unexpectedly during the first night after birth even while feeling happy.

The Postpartum Uterus

Your uterus immediately after delivery still weighs approximately 1 kilogram. During pregnancy it expanded from the size of a pear to an organ capable of holding: a baby, placenta, amniotic fluid, and nearly 5 litres of total contents. Now it must shrink back. This process is called involution. You will feel uterine contractions after birth especially while breastfeeding. These are called afterpains.

They happen because oxytocin released during feeding causes the uterus to contract strongly. For first-time mothers, afterpains are usually mild. For women with previous pregnancies, they can be surprisingly painful. These contractions are beneficial. They: reduce bleeding, compress blood vessels,and help the uterus return to pre-pregnancy size.

My NOTE

Many mothers become frightened the first time they feel abdominal cramping during breastfeeding after delivery. They think something is wrong. In reality, it is evidence that the body is healing correctly. The same hormone helping milk flow to the baby is simultaneously helping the uterus protect the mother from hemorrhage. Human physiology is deeply efficient.

Bleeding After Delivery : What Is Normal

After birth, vaginal bleeding called lochia begins.

Lochia is not simply “leftover blood.” It contains: blood, placental tissue, mucus, inflammatory cells, and uterine lining. It changes over time: Lochia rubra: bright red bleeding in the first days Lochia serosa: pinkish-brown discharge over the next weeks Lochia alba: pale yellow-white discharge toward the end. Bleeding is usually heaviest in the first few days and gradually decreases over 4–6 weeks. Small clots can be normal. However, soaking pads rapidly, very large clots, dizziness, or continuous heavy bleeding requires urgent medical review.

The First Walk to the Bathroom

This moment deserves mention because no one warns women about it properly. Standing up for the first time after delivery can feel shocking. You may feel: weak, shaky, swollen, sore, dizzy, or strangely disconnected from your own body. If you had a vaginal delivery, the perineum may feel bruised or burning. If you had stitches, sitting may hurt. If you had a cesarean section, abdominal movement may feel almost impossible initially. And yet slowly, carefully, the body begins recovering almost immediately.

Your circulation adjusts. Your muscles respond. Your organs begin returning toward their previous positions.

Recovery starts on day one, even when you cannot yet feel it.

THE SCIENCE BEHIND IT

Why Postpartum Sweating Happens

Many women wake drenched in sweat during the first postpartum week.This is normal.

During pregnancy, the body retains large amounts of fluid under the influence of hormones like estrogen and aldosterone. After delivery, this excess fluid must be eliminated. The body does this through: increased urination, and heavy sweating, especially at night. This is one reason postpartum mothers often feel constantly thirsty.

The First Night Feed

Night feeding on the first night is often chaotic. The baby may: latch repeatedly, cluster feed, fall asleep after seconds, cry unpredictably, or seem hungry continuously. This does not mean you are "not producing enough milk."

In the first days: the stomach is tiny, colostrum volume is naturally low, and frequent feeding is biologically designed to stimulate mature milk production. Cluster feeding is not failure. It is endocrine programming.

Every suck sends signals through nerves in the nipple to the hypothalamus and pituitary gland, increasing prolactin and oxytocin release. Your baby is helping build your milk supply.

Emotionally, however, the first night can feel overwhelming.

Many mothers think:

"I don't know what I'm doing."

"The nurses make it look easier."

"What if I cannot do this properly?"

These thoughts are almost universal.

Nobody feels fully prepared the first night they become responsible for a newborn human being.

Your Partner That Night

The first night changes fathers too. Many partners experience:

Helplessness, protectiveness, emotional overload, fear of harming the baby, and deep admiration for the mother. Some become intensely practical, checking blankets, counting feeds, adjusting pillows repeatedly. Others become unusually quiet. This is also normal.

Parenthood reorganises identity for both people, though not always in the same way or at the same speed.

One of the most important things a partner can do during this period is protect the mother's recovery: limiting exhausting visitors, helping with positioning the baby, bringing water and food, monitoring medications, and reminding her that healing takes time.

WHAT YOU MIGHT BE FEELING

Perineal pain or abdominal pain. Heavy fatigue mixed with inability to sleep. Sudden crying spells. Intense attachment to the baby. Fear that something bad might happen if you fall asleep

Hunger is unlike anything experienced during pregnancy. Swelling in hands, legs, or face. Relief that labour is over. Anxiety about taking the baby home. Emotional vulnerability unlike any previous experience.

" The First Night

At 3 a.m., Anjali called the nurse and whispered, embarrassed, "I think the baby is making strange noises."

The nurse picked up the newborn, listened for a few seconds, smiled gently, and said, "That is called breathing." Anjali burst into tears from exhaustion. The nurse sat beside her for a moment and said quietly, "Every mother thinks she is doing it wrong on the first night. Then one day she becomes the person another new mother asks for advice."

Your Body After Delivery

The Healing Nobody Describes Properly

The first time you stand in front of a mirror after delivery, you may not recognise yourself immediately.

Not because you are unrecognisable, but because the body in front of you belongs to someone who has crossed through something immense.

Your abdomen is softer now. Your breasts feel heavy and unfamiliar. There may be swelling in your face, your hands, your feet. Your skin carries marks and shadows that were not there months ago. You may still look pregnant. You may look exhausted in a way sleep alone cannot fix.

And somewhere nearby, usually sleeping with astonishing indifference after having completely transformed your life, is your baby.

This period, the first days and weeks after birth: is one of the most physiologically demanding transitions in human biology. Yet women are often expected to move through it quietly, gracefully, and without complaint. Visitors arrive carrying flowers and opinions. Phones fill with messages asking for baby photographs. Relatives ask whether the baby is feeding well, sleeping well, gaining weight well.

Very few people ask the mother how her body feels.

The truth is that postpartum recovery is not a single event. It is a slow reconstruction. Pregnancy altered almost every organ system in your body, and after delivery, each of those systems must gradually find its way back toward equilibrium.

Immediately after birth, your uterus is still enormous. During pregnancy it expanded from the size of a small pear to an organ capable of holding a full-grown baby, placenta, and litres of amniotic fluid. After delivery, it does not instantly disappear back into the pelvis. In the first days postpartum, you can often still feel it firmly beneath your abdomen, sitting approximately at the level of the navel. And then, quietly and steadily, it begins shrinking. This process is called involution. It is one of the most extraordinary examples of physiological healing in medicine.

Over approximately six weeks, the uterus contracts day after day, reducing from nearly one kilogram in weight back toward its non-pregnant size of around sixty to eighty grams.

You may feel these contractions unexpectedly while breastfeeding. A sharp tightening across the lower abdomen. A cramp that briefly steals your breath. Many women become frightened the first time this happens, assuming something is wrong. In reality, it is evidence that the body is healing exactly as it should.

Oxytocin — the same hormone responsible for milk let-down and emotional bonding — is causing the uterus to contract firmly, compressing blood vessels and protecting the mother from postpartum hemorrhage. The body, remarkably, is nourishing the baby and saving the mother simultaneously. There is also the bleeding.

No one truly prepares women for how long postpartum bleeding lasts. After delivery, the uterus sheds blood, mucus, inflammatory cells, and residual placental tissue in a discharge called lochia. In the beginning it is bright red and surprisingly heavy, more like a prolonged menstrual period than the delicate spotting many women imagine. Gradually it becomes pinkish-brown, then pale yellow-white over the following weeks.

This is not simply "leftover blood." It is the internal surface of the uterus healing itself after the placenta detached from its wall.

And while all this is happening internally, the outside of the body is healing too.

If you delivered vaginally, your perineum may feel bruised, swollen, and intensely tender. Sitting can become an engineering problem requiring pillows, careful positioning, and patience. Passing urine may sting. Even walking may feel unfamiliar for several days. Women who required stitches often describe a strange pulling sensation, a persistent awareness of the body in a place they had never consciously noticed before labour.

And yet, despite the discomfort, healing begins immediately. Blood flow increases to damaged tissues. Swelling slowly decreases. New collagen forms. Pain that feels overwhelming on day two often becomes manageable by the second week.

Women recovering from cesarean section experience a different but equally significant healing process. A cesarean is major abdominal surgery, though society has an unfortunate tendency to discuss it casually. Skin, fascia, abdominal muscles, and uterus have all been surgically opened and repaired. The mother is simultaneously recovering from surgery and adapting to newborn care. The first time she tries to sit up alone after surgery can feel almost impossible.

Laughing hurts. Coughing hurts. Turning in bed hurts. Even holding the baby for long periods may strain exhausted abdominal muscles. And yet many women still apologise for needing help. They should not. Recovery after cesarean birth deserves the same seriousness and compassion as recovery after any major operation. Then there is the abdomen itself, perhaps the part of postpartum recovery women think about most and speak about least honestly. Many women expect the stomach to flatten after delivery because the baby is gone. Instead they discover a soft, swollen abdomen that still resembles pregnancy. This surprises them, even embarrasses them sometimes, particularly in a world obsessed with rapid "bounce-back" culture. But biologically, nothing about immediate recovery is designed to look aesthetically finished. The uterus is still enlarged. The abdominal muscles are stretched. The skin has lost tension temporarily. Fluid remains trapped within tissues. Internal organs are gradually shifting back toward their original positions.

Healing does not happen overnight because pregnancy did not happen overnight. For some women, the abdominal muscles themselves separate during pregnancy under the pressure of the growing uterus. This condition, diastasis recti, leaves a soft weakness through the centre of the abdomen that can persist postpartum. Women may notice a bulge while sitting up or a feeling of poor core strength that simple exercise does not immediately fix. This is not failure. It is anatomy responding to extraordinary mechanical stress. The postpartum body also leaks constantly in ways no one adequately warns women about.

Milk leaks through bras and bedsheets. Sweat soaks clothes at night as the body eliminates excess pregnancy fluid. Urine may escape unexpectedly while laughing or coughing because pelvic floor muscles are exhausted from months of pressure and childbirth itself.

Even hair changes. During pregnancy, high estrogen levels prolong the growth phase of hair, making it feel thick and glossy. After delivery, estrogen falls dramatically and many hairs enter the shedding phase simultaneously. Around three months postpartum, women often panic as hair begins falling in handfuls during showers and combing. But this too is temporary. The body is recalibrating itself hormonally after one of the largest endocrine shifts it will ever experience. And through all this healing, the mother is expected to nurture another human being continuously. She feeds while sore. Sleeps while alert. Recovers while giving. That is the part of postpartum physiology textbooks rarely capture properly: recovery after childbirth is not rest. It is active healing under conditions of profound sleep deprivation and constant biological demand.

My NOTE

I sometimes think the postpartum body deserves more admiration than the pregnant body, because pregnancy still carries anticipation and celebration around it. Postpartum recovery happens more quietly. The world's attention shifts toward the baby, while the mother continues healing in the background.

But I have watched women survive major blood loss, surgery, sleeplessness, pain, fear, breastfeeding difficulties, hormonal storms, and overwhelming responsibility, all while continuing to care for a newborn with astonishing tenderness.

The postpartum body is not weak. It is one of the strongest things medicine ever witnesses. There comes a moment, usually weeks later, when a mother catches sight of herself unexpectedly in a mirror and realises something important. She does not look exactly like the woman she was before pregnancy. But she does not need to.

Because this body now carries evidence of transformation, survival, and creation.

Breastfeeding

The Learning Curve Nobody Warns You About

There is a particular kind of silence that exists at 2 a.m. when a mother is sitting upright in bed trying to feed a crying newborn for the fourth time in one night.

The room is dark except for a dim lamp. Her hair is tied hurriedly. Her body still aches from delivery. One breast is leaking through her shirt while the baby struggles to latch onto the other. Somewhere nearby, untouched food has gone cold. She is exhausted enough to cry, but too tired to actually do it.

And in that moment, almost every new mother thinks the same thing:

"Everyone said breastfeeding was natural. Why does this feel so difficult?" The answer is important. Breastfeeding is natural. But natural things are not always instinctively easy. Walking is natural too, but babies still fall repeatedly before learning it. Breastfeeding is a biological process that requires coordination between two people who have never done this together before — a newborn learning to feed and a mother learning to nourish.

Both are beginners. One of the most damaging myths surrounding breastfeeding is the idea that it should happen perfectly and effortlessly from the very first feed. When reality turns out to be more complicated, painful latching, crying babies, uncertainty about milk supply, exhaustion, many mothers assume they are failing. They are not failing. They are learning.

The First Milk

For the first few days after delivery, your breasts produce colostrum rather than mature milk. Colostrum is thick, concentrated, yellow-golden in colour, and produced in surprisingly small amounts. Many mothers become anxious because they expect milk to flow immediately in large quantities. Instead they see only drops. Those drops are enough.

A newborn stomach on the first day of life is extraordinarily small roughly the size of a cherry. Colostrum is designed perfectly for that stomach. It is rich in protein, antibodies, immune cells, and growth factors that line and protect the newborn intestine.

Scientifically, colostrum functions almost like the baby's first vaccine.

It contains particularly high levels of secretory IgA, an antibody that coats the infant gut and reduces the risk of infection while the newborn immune system is still immature. It also helps establish the early microbiome, the complex bacterial ecosystem that will influence digestion, metabolism, and immunity for years to come. The body has prepared this milk specifically for the first days of life. Nothing about it is inadequate.

YOUR BABY RIGHT NOW Two to five days old.

Your baby is still adapting to the outside world. Feeding is not only about nutrition yet. It is also about regulation. Feeding stabilises blood sugar, temperature, breathing, and emotional security. Newborns often want to remain attached to the breast not simply because they are hungry, but because feeding regulates almost every physiological system in their bodies.

This is why babies sometimes feed again only thirty minutes after a long feed. It does not necessarily mean the previous feed "was not enough." Sometimes the baby is seeking warmth, regulation, comfort, or neurological calmness in addition to milk. When Milk "Comes In" Around the third to fifth day postpartum, many mothers wake up and realise something dramatic has changed overnight.

The breasts feel: swollen, hot, heavy, tight, almost painfully full.

This transition is commonly described as milk "coming in," though technically milk production began much earlier. What is happening now is a rapid increase in mature milk volume triggered by hormonal shifts after delivery of the placenta.

Progesterone levels fall sharply after birth. In response, prolactin begins driving large-scale milk synthesis within the breast tissue.

The breasts become engorged partly because of milk accumulation and partly because of increased blood flow and lymphatic fluid.

Some women describe this sensation as fullness. Others describe it as feeling "like rocks attached to the chest."

Both descriptions are medically understandable.

The body at this stage is still learning supply regulation. Frequent feeding helps establish balance between milk production and milk removal. This early period is biologically sensitive. The breasts are essentially interpreting the baby's feeding behaviour as instructions:

feed frequently → produce more milk,

feed less frequently → reduce supply.

The newborn and maternal endocrine system are building a communication pattern together.

The Latch

A good latch changes everything. A poor latch can make breastfeeding physically miserable. Many mothers imagine breastfeeding pain is inevitable. Mild tenderness initially can be normal, but severe pain, cracked nipples, bleeding, or curling your toes in agony every time the baby feeds usually indicates positioning or latch problems rather than "weakness" on the mother's part. A properly latched baby takes not only the nipple into the mouth but a large portion of the areola beneath it. The baby's mouth should appear wide open, lips flanged outward, chin pressed into the breast, with rhythmic deep swallowing rather than rapid shallow sucking.

When the latch is correct: feeding becomes more efficient, milk transfer improves, nipples heal, and the baby remains satisfied longer. When it is not correct: the baby swallows air, feeds continuously without satisfaction, and the mother becomes progressively injured and exhausted. This is why skilled lactation support matters enormously in the early days.

My NOTE

I wish more women understood this: struggling with breastfeeding initially does not mean you are a bad mother, an incapable woman, or "not made for breastfeeding." It means you are postpartum. You are exhausted. Hormonal. Healing. Learning. Sleep deprived. And trying to feed a human being who also has absolutely no idea what they are doing yet.

Please be gentler with yourself during this period. The Emotional Weight of Feeding. Few parts of early motherhood carry as much emotional pressure as infant feeding. Women are told: breast is best, exclusive breastfeeding is ideal, formula should be avoided, good mothers persist.

All of which, in simplified form, may be medically true. But what often gets lost is compassion for the mother herself. A woman recovering from traumatic delivery, severe pain, hemorrhage, surgery, depression, prematurity, or a medically complicated newborn experience may find breastfeeding emotionally overwhelming. Some women breastfeed easily and joyfully. Some work very hard to establish it. Some partially breastfeed. Some cannot breastfeed despite desperately wanting to. Some choose not to continue. None of these situations erase maternal love.

Medicine should support breastfeeding strongly while also protecting maternal mental health with equal seriousness.

Cluster Feeding — Why Babies Suddenly Feed Constantly

One evening, usually around the second or third week, many mothers become convinced something has gone terribly wrong.

The baby suddenly wants to feed: every thirty minutes, for hours, while crying if removed from the breast. This is called cluster feeding. It is exhausting. It is biologically normal. Cluster feeding often occurs during: growth spurts, evening fussiness, developmental transitions, and periods of increased milk-demand signalling. The baby is not "using you as a pacifier." The baby is increasing supply through repeated stimulation. Human milk production is demand-driven physiology.

However, understanding the science does not automatically make cluster feeding emotionally easier at midnight after four hours of broken sleep. This is where support matters. A mother should not be expected to survive early postpartum entirely alone.

The Partner's Role in Breastfeeding

Partners often feel helpless during breastfeeding because they cannot physically feed the baby themselves.

But successful breastfeeding frequently depends on non-feeding support: bringing water,preparing meals, helping position pillows, burping the baby afterward, changing diapers at night, protecting the mother from excessive visitors, and noticing when she is emotionally overwhelmed. One of the strongest predictors of breastfeeding continuation is not maternal "willpower." It is practical support.

THE SCIENCE BEHIND IT

Why Breastfeeding Makes You Sleepy

Oxytocin released during breastfeeding has calming neurological effects. It lowers stress hormone activity and promotes relaxation and bonding.

Prolactin; the hormone responsible for milk production, also has sedative properties. This is one reason many mothers become intensely sleepy during night feeds. Human physiology is trying to encourage rest whenever possible, even in fragmented sleep conditions. And Then There Is the Guilt Perhaps the hardest part of infant feeding is not always the physical difficulty. Sometimes it is the guilt. Guilt if breastfeeding hurts. Guilt if the baby loses weight. Guilt if formula is needed temporarily. Guilt if pumping feels exhausting. Guilt if breastfeeding continues. Guilt if breastfeeding stops. Motherhood has a way of convincing women that every decision carries enormous moral significance.

But babies do not need morally perfect mothers.

They need: responsive mothers, emotionally available mothers, supported mothers, recovering mothers, mothers allowed to remain human.

WHAT YOU MIGHT BE FEELING

The early breastfeeding weeks often contain contradictory emotions existing simultaneously. Pride and exhaustion. Deep attachment and resentment at constant physical demand. Confidence during one feed and panic during the next. Many mothers feel emotionally overwhelmed precisely because feeding is so constant. The body no longer entirely belongs to itself, and adapting to that reality takes time.

There are moments when feeding feels peaceful and almost sacred — the quiet weight of a sleeping baby against your chest, tiny fingers opening and closing against your skin.

And there are moments when you desperately want uninterrupted sleep more than anything else in the world.

Both experiences can exist together in the same mother.

" Asha's Third Night

On the third night after delivery, Asha sat crying softly while her baby screamed at her breast. "I think he hates me," she whispered when I entered the room. She had not slept properly in nearly four days. Her nipples were cracked. Her milk had just started coming in and her breasts were painfully engorged.

The baby was hungry. The mother was frightened. Both were exhausted. The nurse helped reposition the baby slightly, chin deeper against the breast, mouth wider, body turned fully toward the mother. Within seconds, the crying stopped. The baby began swallowing rhythmically. Asha looked down in stunned silence and then burst into tears again, this time from relief. Years later she told me, laughing, "I genuinely thought motherhood had ended on day three."

The Emotional Storm of the First Week

When Happiness and Exhaustion Live Together. There is a moment in the first week after birth when many mothers realise something deeply confusing: They are happy.

And overwhelmed, grateful, frightened, completely exhausted. All at the same time.

This emotional contradiction surprises people because society speaks about motherhood in extremes. Women are taught to expect either glowing bliss or obvious depression, profound joy or obvious suffering. In reality, the early postpartum period is usually far more emotionally complex than either stereotype allows.

You may spend one hour staring at your baby with overwhelming love so intense it physically hurts. And the next hour crying because someone asked what you wanted for breakfast. This does not mean something is wrong with you. It means your brain, body, hormones, identity, sleep cycle, relationships, and nervous system are all being reorganised simultaneously. The first postpartum week is not simply recovery from delivery. It is neurological and emotional reconstruction.

The Hormonal Collapse After Birth

Pregnancy hormones rise gradually over months. After delivery, they fall with astonishing speed. Within hours after the placenta is delivered, estrogen levels drop dramatically. Progesterone collapses. Oxytocin fluctuates with feeding and physical closeness. Prolactin rises. Cortisol patterns change. Thyroid function shifts. Neurotransmitter systems begin recalibrating.

Few endocrine transitions in medicine are as sudden as the postpartum hormonal shift. And hormones do not simply influence reproduction. They influence mood, sleep, appetite, emotional regulation, memory, anxiety, stress response, and cognition itself. This is why many women feel emotionally fragile during the first week even when everything medically appears normal.

YOUR BODY RIGHT NOW

During the first postpartum week, your nervous system remains in a state of heightened vigilance. Sleep deprivation begins impairing concentration and emotional buffering. Oxytocin surges repeatedly during skin-to-skin contact and feeding, intensifying attachment and emotional sensitivity simultaneously. Your brain becomes biologically tuned toward infant monitoring, which is why many mothers wake instantly at tiny newborn sounds while sleeping through everything else.

The postpartum maternal brain is not weaker than before pregnancy. It is differently prioritised.

The Baby Blues

Approximately seventy to eighty percent of mothers experience what is commonly called the “baby blues” during the first week postpartum. The name sounds trivial. The experience often does not. Baby blues usually begin around day three to five postpartum, exactly when milk comes in, sleep deprivation worsens, physical pain accumulates, and hormones fluctuate most dramatically.

Women describe crying unexpectedly, feeling emotionally sensitive, becoming irritable, overwhelmed, anxious without clear reason, or suddenly sad despite loving the baby deeply. One minute they are fine. The next minute they are crying because the baby yawned. This emotional instability can feel frightening if no one has explained it beforehand. But baby blues are generally temporary and self-limiting. They usually improve within two weeks as hormones stabilise and the mother gradually adapts physically and emotionally to postpartum life.

What matters is understanding the difference between normal emotional vulnerability and postpartum depression. The Difference Between Baby Blues and Postpartum Depression. Baby blues fluctuate. Postpartum depression persists. A mother with baby blues usually still experiences moments of pleasure, humour, relief, or emotional connection between emotional waves.

Postpartum depression is deeper, heavier, and more continuous.

Symptoms may include persistent hopelessness, emotional numbness, inability to bond with the baby, severe guilt, panic, loss of appetite, insomnia even when exhausted, intrusive thoughts, or thoughts of self-harm.

This is not weakness. It is not failure. It is not "bad motherhood."

Postpartum depression is a genuine medical condition involving biological, psychological, and social factors. And it is treatable.

My NOTE

One of the most dangerous myths in motherhood is the belief that loving your baby should automatically make postpartum emotionally easy. I have seen deeply loving mothers struggle profoundly after delivery. Love does not protect the nervous system from sleep deprivation, hormonal collapse, surgical recovery, physical pain, isolation, anxiety, or depression. Sometimes women believe that because they wanted the baby very much, they have no right to struggle afterward. They do have that right. The Mental Weight of Responsibility. Pregnancy carries anticipation. Motherhood carries responsibility.

Suddenly another human being depends on you continuously

for feeding, warmth, regulation, comfort, and survival itself. The psychological weight of this responsibility arrives immediately after birth.

Many mothers become hypervigilant in the first week. They repeatedly check whether the baby is breathing. They wake suddenly in panic. They imagine accidents. They feel unable to relax fully even when someone else is holding the baby.

This behaviour is partly psychological and partly biological. The maternal brain becomes highly sensitive to infant-related stimuli after delivery. Functional MRI studies show increased activation in emotional processing and vigilance centres when mothers hear their own babies cry.

You are not becoming irrational. Your brain is adapting toward protection. Sleep Deprivation Changes Everything No discussion of the first postpartum week is complete without acknowledging sleep deprivation honestly.

Broken sleep affects emotional regulation, pain tolerance, memory, patience, milk supply, anxiety, and perception itself.

After several nights of fragmented sleep, even small difficulties can feel catastrophic. A crying baby at three in the morning feels very different to an exhausted brain than it does at three in the afternoon.

This is why postpartum support matters so profoundly. Human beings were never biologically designed to recover from childbirth and raise newborns in complete isolation. Throughout most of human history, mothers were surrounded by sisters, grandmothers, neighbours, and shared caregiving structures.

Modern motherhood often expects recovery inside emotional and physical isolation while simultaneously presenting impossible standards through social media and cultural pressure. The result is predictable exhaustion.

The Strange Loneliness of New Motherhood

Even deeply loved mothers can feel lonely postpartum.

Visitors come briefly and leave. Partners return to work. Conversations narrow around feeding schedules and diapers. The outside world continues normally while your entire existence revolves around two-hour intervals. Many women describe feeling as though time itself has changed after birth.

Days blur. Nights stretch endlessly. Meals become fragmented. The body no longer belongs fully to itself. Privacy disappears. And yet simultaneously, mothers may feel guilty for missing aspects of their previous lives because they love the baby so much

Contradictory emotions coexist constantly in early motherhood.

THE SCIENCE BEHIND IT

Why Mothers Become Emotionally Sensitive to Crying. Newborn crying activates multiple regions in the maternal brain associated with threat detection, emotional processing, empathy, motor planning, and hormonal response. Oxytocin and prolactin increase responsiveness to infant distress signals, making mothers biologically more reactive to crying than most other adults.

This heightened sensitivity improves infant survival. It also contributes to maternal emotional exhaustion. Your Relationship With Your Partner. The first week after birth changes relationships immediately. Couples who functioned smoothly before delivery may suddenly find themselves irritable, sleep deprived, emotionally reactive, and struggling to communicate clearly. Tiny disagreements become amplified through exhaustion. One partner may feel physically overwhelmed. The other may feel helpless or excluded. Both may feel unprepared.

This does not mean the relationship is damaged. It means both people are adapting simultaneously under conditions of stress and sleep deprivation. Gentleness matters enormously during this phase. So does practical teamwork. Sometimes the most loving postpartum gestures are surprisingly ordinary: bringing water without being asked, taking the baby for thirty minutes, changing a diaper during the night, or saying “you’re doing well” at exactly the right moment.

The Identity Shift

Perhaps the deepest emotional change of the first postpartum week is invisible. A woman who has spent her entire life being someone's daughter, student, partner, professional, and friend suddenly realises another human being now knows her primarily as mother. Identity shifts rarely happen all at once psychologically, even though they happen instantly socially.

Some women feel maternal immediately. Some grow into motherhood gradually. Some feel disconnected at first and terrified to admit it. All of these experiences exist within normal human emotional range.Motherhood is not always a lightning strike. Sometimes it is a slow sunrise.

WHAT YOU MIGHT BE FEELING

The first week postpartum often feels emotionally disproportionate. Small comments hurt more than expected. Kindness feels overwhelming. Fatigue magnifies everything. You may cry while feeding the baby and then laugh minutes later at something absurdly small. Many mothers feel simultaneously stronger and more fragile than they have ever felt before.

There are moments of astonishing tenderness during this week.And moments when you stare at the clock at four in the morning wondering how human beings survive early parenthood at allBoth belong to the same story.

" Kavya's Sixth Day

On the sixth day after delivery, Kavya sat holding her sleeping daughter and crying silently. "I think something is wrong with me," she whispered. "I wanted this baby so much. Why am I crying every day?" Her mother, who had quietly been folding tiny baby clothes nearby, answered before I could. "Because you have just crossed from one life into another," she said softly. "No woman crosses something that large without tears." Kavya later told me that sentence stayed with her longer than any medical advice she received postpartum.

Sleep, Healing, and Survival

The Weeks That Feel Endless and Pass Too Quickly. In the early weeks after birth, time behaves strangely. Days feel impossibly long. Nights feel even longer. And yet somehow, when mothers look back later, the entire period seems blurred together into one continuous stretch of feeding, holding, waking, soothing, and surviving. This is the phase of motherhood few people describe honestly enough. Pregnancy has ended. Visitors have mostly stopped coming. The congratulatory messages slow down. Partners often return to work. The house gradually becomes quieter. And inside that quietness begins the real work of early parenthood. A newborn does not understand day and night. Hunger arrives every two to three hours with biological urgency. Feeding sessions merge into diaper changes, burping, rocking, washing clothes, trying to sleep, and beginning again.

Many mothers describe the early postpartum weeks not as individual days but as cycles.

Feed, Burp, Settle, Sleep briefly, Wake again....Repeat.

And while all this is happening externally, the mother's body is still healing internally with astonishing intensity.

The Myth of "Resting After Delivery"

People often say postpartum women should "rest." This is medically correct and practically absurd at the same time. True rest after childbirth is difficult because recovery occurs alongside continuous infant care. Even when the baby sleeps, the mother may still be:feeding,pumping,bleeding, bathing, changing clothes, trying to eat, replying to relatives, or lying awake listening for the baby to breathe. Sleep after childbirth becomes fragmented into short intervals rather than long restorative stretches. And fragmented sleep affects nearly every system in the body.

YOUR BODY RIGHT NOW

Two to six weeks postpartum.

Your uterus is continuing involution. Hormone levels remain unstable. Blood volume is normalising. Breast tissue is adjusting dynamically to feeding demand. Pelvic floor muscles are healing. Tissue repair is ongoing at both microscopic and muscular levels. Meanwhile, chronic sleep interruption is affecting emotional regulation, immune function, metabolism, and pain perception.

Healing is still actively happening, even if the outside world has begun expecting normal functioning again.

Why Sleep Deprivation Feels So Extreme

Newborn sleep biology is fundamentally different from adult sleep biology. A newborn wakes frequently because: stomach capacity is tiny, blood sugar reserves are limited, neurological development is immature, and frequent feeding protects survival.

This waking pattern is biologically normal.

Unfortunately, what is biologically normal for newborns can be physically devastating for adults. Interrupted sleep prevents the brain from completing normal restorative cycles. Over time, this affects: concentration, memory, emotional, resilience, decision-making, patience and physical recovery.

This is why postpartum mothers sometimes: cry unexpectedly, forget simple things, feel emotionally overwhelmed, become unusually irritable, or feel detached from reality after difficult nights. Sleep deprivation is not laziness. It is neurophysiology.

My NOTE

One of the most harmful expectations placed on new mothers is the idea that they should continue functioning normally despite severe sleep deprivation. If an exhausted surgeon, pilot, or doctor began forgetting words, crying unexpectedly, and struggling to think clearly after sleeping in two-hour intervals for weeks, everyone would recognise it as physiological exhaustion. But postpartum mothers are expected to continue smiling through it quietly. They deserve far more understanding than they usually receive.

The Night Feeds

There is a specific loneliness to feeding a baby in the middle of the night. The rest of the world is asleep. The house is dark. Outside, everything appears calm and silent while inside your body and home an enormous amount of work is happening.

Many mothers remember these feeds vividly years later:

the weight of the baby against their chest, the dim yellow light, the strange stillness of 3 a.m., the exhaustion is so deep it almost feels unreal.

Night feeds are physically demanding partly because prolactin levels rise naturally during nighttime hours, increasing milk production. From a biological perspective, human lactation is designed around frequent night feeding.

This is efficient for infant survival. It is considerably less efficient for maternal sleep. And yet many mothers later remember these nights with unexpected tenderness because intimacy grows quietly during repetitive care. Attachment is often built not during dramatic moments, but during ordinary exhausted ones repeated thousands of times.

The Body's Quiet Recovery

One of the remarkable things about postpartum healing is how much recovery happens invisibly.

Every day: the uterus becomes slightly smaller, blood vessels heal, hormone patterns stabilize, inflammation decreases, muscles regain tone, surgical wounds strengthen, nerves repair themselves, and the cardiovascular system recalibrates.

But because these changes happen gradually, mothers often feel as though nothing is improving. Healing rarely feels dramatic while it is happening. It simply accumulates slowly until one day a woman realises: she walked without pain, laughed without holding her abdomen, slept for four consecutive hours, or looked in the mirror and recognised herself again.

Recovery is usually noticed backward rather than forward.

The Pressure to "Enjoy Every Moment" New mothers are often told: "Enjoy every moment." "They grow so fast." "You'll miss this phase." These statements are usually well intentioned.

But to an exhausted postpartum woman recovering physically while functioning on fragmented sleep, they can feel strangely guilt-inducing. Because the truth is: some moments are beautiful, and some moments are simply hard.

You can love your baby deeply and still hate waking up six times overnight. You can feel grateful and exhausted simultaneously.

You can miss your previous freedom while also not wanting a single second away from your child. Human emotion is capable of contradiction. Motherhood does not erase that complexity.

THE SCIENCE BEHIND IT

Why Newborns Prefer Being Held

Inside the uterus, the baby existed in constant motion, warmth, pressure, and sound. The maternal heartbeat, breathing movements, walking, voice, and abdominal compression created a continuously regulated sensory environment. After birth, sudden separation into quiet flat surfaces can feel neurologically unfamiliar to newborns.

This is why babies often sleep better: on a parent's chest, while being carried, or during movement. Contact regulates infant heart rate, breathing, temperature, and stress hormone activity.

Your baby is not "becoming spoiled" by wanting closeness. Your baby is adapting to existence outside the womb. Visitors, Advice, and Overstimulation By the second or third postpartum week, many mothers begin feeling emotionally overloaded by advice.

Everyone has opinions:
- how often the baby should feed,
- whether the baby is cold,
- whether the mother should eat certain foods,
- whether the baby is sleeping correctly,
- *whether the mother is holding the baby too much or too little.*

Much of this advice comes from love. But postpartum women are highly emotionally sensitive, physically tired, and cognitively overloaded. Constant criticism or conflicting advice can become psychologically exhausting very quickly.

A recovering mother does not need perfection. She needs: reassurance, practical support, nourishment, hydration, rest, and protection from unnecessary stress.

The Small Survival Strategies

In medicine, survival is sometimes built from small interventions repeated consistently. The same is true postpartum. Women cope better when they: sleep whenever support is available, eat regularly instead of waiting until starving, accept help, reduce unnecessary visitors, shower daily if possible, spend brief periods outdoors, and speak honestly about emotional difficulty.

Tiny acts of care matter enormously during recovery. So does hearing the sentence: "You are allowed to find this hard."

The Couple During Survival Mode

Early parenthood often transforms relationships temporarily into logistical partnerships. Conversations become:
"Did the baby feed?"
"Where are the wipes?"
"When did you last sleep?"
"Can you hold him while I shower?"

Romance may feel distant for a while.This is normal.

Intimacy after childbirth often changes before it returns. Physical recovery, hormonal shifts, exhaustion, breastfeeding, and identity changes all influence desire and emotional connection. Couples who survive this period best are rarely the couples who remain perfectly calm. They are usually the couples who remain kind during exhaustion.That matters more.

WHAT YOU MIGHT BE FEELING

By the second or third postpartum week, many mothers begin experiencing emotional whiplash between increasing confidence and increasing exhaustion. You may feel more capable caring for the baby while simultaneously feeling more depleted physically. Some days feel manageable. Others feel impossible for reasons you cannot fully explain.

You may suddenly miss ordinary things: uninterrupted sleep, hot tea, silence, your previous routine, your previous body, spontaneous freedom.Missing those things does not reduce maternal love. It simply means you are still human beneath the role of mother. And gradually, almost invisibly, survival begins becoming adaptation.

" Rhea's Fourth Week

At four weeks postpartum, Rhea told me quietly, "I think I finally understand why new mothers cry when someone brings them food." She had spent the previous month functioning in fragments of sleep, feeding constantly, recovering from stitches, and trying to appear grateful and capable at all times.

"One afternoon my neighbour came over with hot dal and fresh rotis," she said. "She didn't ask to hold the baby. She didn't give advice. She just said, 'Eat while it's hot,' and left."

Rhea laughed softly afterward. "I nearly fell in love with her."

Your Relationship After Baby

Loving Each Other While Learning Parenthood. A baby enters a family quietly at first. One small bassinet beside the bed. Tiny clothes drying near the window. Feeding schedules written on scraps of paper. Soft crying in the middle of the night. And yet despite that physical smallness, nothing alters a relationship more completely than the arrival of a child.

Before the baby, love existed primarily between two people. After the baby, love becomes divided, redistributed, exhausted, protective, logistical, physical, hormonal, and sometimes unexpectedly fragile. Most couples are unprepared for how dramatic this transition feels.

Not because the relationship is weak. But because early parenthood places two sleep-deprived human beings under continuous emotional and physical strain while simultaneously demanding they care for another completely dependent life. Even strong relationships feel the pressure.

The Couple Before and After Birth

During pregnancy, couples often imagine parenthood emotionally. They picture: holding the baby, choosing names, taking photographs, decorating rooms, imagining the future.

What they usually do not imagine fully is the relentless practical intensity of newborn care. The first weeks after birth contain: interrupted sleep, physical recovery, hormonal instability, financial anxiety, feeding stress, constant decision-making, and profound exhaustion.

Under those conditions, even ordinary communication becomes difficult. Small disagreements suddenly feel enormous. One partner may feel overwhelmed physically. The other may feel helpless emotionally. Both may secretly believe the other is coping better.This misunderstanding is extremely common.

YOUR LIFE RIGHT NOW

Your household is reorganising itself around survival and adaptation. Routines that once felt automatic no longer exist. Sleep, intimacy, meals, conversations, and personal space have all changed simultaneously. Both partners are grieving certain aspects of their previous lives while also loving the child who caused those changes. This emotional contradiction is not relationship failure.It is transition.

The Mother's Experience

After childbirth, many women feel emotionally transformed faster than their partners. This is partly psychological and partly biological. Pregnancy, labour, breastfeeding, and postpartum hormonal changes create an intense physical immersion into motherhood from the very beginning. A mother's body becomes the centre of feeding, soothing, recovery, and infant regulation immediately after birth. Meanwhile, her identity changes overnight. Suddenly: her body no longer entirely belongs to her, privacy becomes limited, physical exhaustion becomes constant, and everyone around her focuses primarily on the baby.

Many women quietly begin feeling invisible during this period.
People ask:
"How is the baby sleeping?"
"Is the baby feeding well?"
"Has the baby gained weight?"

Very few ask: "How are you coping emotionally?" This invisibility can create loneliness even inside loving relationships.

The Partner's Experience

Partners often experience a quieter but equally significant transition. Many fathers describe: feeling protective, emotionally overwhelmed, frightened of making mistakes, unsure how to help, or excluded from the intense mother-baby bond during breastfeeding.

Some become intensely practical, focusing on finances, routines, supplies, and logistics because action feels easier than vulnerability. Others feel helpless watching the mother struggle physically and emotionally without being able to "fix" the situation.And because attention shifts heavily toward the baby and recovering mother, partners sometimes suppress their own emotional adjustment entirely. But parenthood changes both people.Even when the changes happen differently.

My NOTE

One of the strongest predictors of relationship stability after childbirth is not whether couples argue. All couples argue during exhaustion. The real predictor is whether they continue treating each other as allies while arguing.

Early parenthood can make people speak sharply, cry unexpectedly, or withdraw emotionally from sheer fatigue. Couples survive this period best when they remember that the problem is usually exhaustion, not each other.

The Disappearance of Time Together

One of the hardest realities for couples after birth is how suddenly uninterrupted time disappears. Before the baby, conversations happened naturally: during dinner, before sleep, while travelling, during ordinary quiet moments.

After birth, conversations become fragmented between feeds, diaper changes, crying spells, and exhaustion. Many couples realise they have not truly spoken in days except about logistics.

This can feel emotionally frightening. But it is usually temporary.

In early parenthood, relationships often move briefly from romance into survival partnership. That shift can feel unromantic, but it is not unloving. Sometimes love in the postpartum period looks less like passion and more like: reheating food, refilling water bottles, washing pump parts, changing diapers without complaint, or taking the baby so the other person can sleep for ninety uninterrupted minutes. These acts matter enormously.

Physical Intimacy After Birth

Few subjects create more anxiety postpartum than physical intimacy. After delivery, many women feel disconnected from sexuality temporarily because: the body is healing, hormones are changing, estrogen levels are low, breastfeeding suppresses vaginal lubrication, exhaustion is overwhelming, and physical touch has become associated with constant caregiving.

Even women deeply in love with their partners may feel emotionally or physically distant for a period after childbirth. This is normal. The postpartum body is recovering from: labour, bleeding, stitches, surgery, breastfeeding, hormonal collapse, and chronic sleep disruption. Desire often returns gradually rather than suddenly. Pressure during this phase is harmful. Patience is protective. Most medical guidelines recommend waiting until approximately six weeks postpartum before penetrative intercourse, though emotional readiness varies enormously between individuals.Healing is not only physical. It is neurological and emotional too.

THE SCIENCE BEHIND IT

Why Libido Often Changes After Childbirth

Breastfeeding suppresses ovarian estrogen production through elevated prolactin levels. Lower estrogen contributes to: vaginal dryness, reduced libido, and physical discomfort during intercourse. Additionally, chronic sleep deprivation increases cortisol and reduces testosterone levels in both men and women, further affecting sexual desire. From a biological perspective, the postpartum period is hormonally oriented toward infant survival rather than reproduction.

The Resentment Nobody Expects

One of the most difficult emotions couples experience postpartum is resentment. Mothers may resent: unequal sleep, unequal recovery burden, unequal physical sacrifice, or feeling solely responsible for the baby.

Partners may resent: emotional distance, feeling unappreciated, loss of intimacy, or never feeling "good enough" in helping. These feelings often frighten couples because they interpret them as signs of relationship damage. Usually they are signs of exhaustion and unmet needs. Resentment grows fastest where appreciation disappears.

Simple acknowledgment matters more than people realise:
"I know you're tired." "Thank you for doing that." "You're doing well." "I know this is hard."
Tiny sentences can prevent enormous emotional distance.

Protecting the Mother

Across many traditional cultures, postpartum recovery involved structured protection of the mother: reduced workload, family support, nutritional care, restricted visitors, and designated healing periods.

Modern life often removes these protections while keeping expectations high. A recovering mother should not be expected to: host guests, entertain relatives, resume full domestic responsibilities, or function normally immediately after childbirth.Protecting maternal recovery is not indulgence. It is healthcare. And partners play a critical role in that protection.

The New Shape of Love

Perhaps the most surprising thing about parenthood is that love changes shape repeatedly. The love between partners after a baby is often less spontaneous for a while but more deliberate.

You choose each other actively during exhaustion.
You continue showing up despite stress.
You forgive quickly because both people are overwhelmed.
You learn each other again inside new identities.

And occasionally, usually in the middle of complete chaos, there are moments so unexpectedly tender they feel almost unbearable: seeing your partner asleep holding the baby, watching them calm the newborn instinctively, hearing them called "Papa" or "Mama" for the first time. In those moments, couples often realise something profound. The relationship did not disappear after the baby. It transformed.

WHAT YOU MIGHT BE FEELING

The postpartum relationship period often contains emotional contradictions. You may feel deeply connected to your partner one moment and irrationally irritated the next. Exhaustion magnifies misunderstandings while simultaneously making tenderness feel more meaningful than before.

Many couples worry privately during the first months:

"Will we ever feel normal again?" Usually, slowly, the answer becomes yes. Not the old normal. A new one. One built around three people instead of two.

" Nidhi and Aryaa

Three weeks after delivery, Nidhi burst into tears because Arjun had forgotten to buy diapers on his way home.

"I remember thinking our marriage was collapsing over diapers," she later told me, laughing. In reality, both of them were profoundly exhausted. Nidhi was breastfeeding every two hours while recovering from stitches. Arjun had returned to work while sleeping in fragments and worrying constantly about finances and the baby. That night, after the baby finally slept, Arjun quietly said, "I think we are both drowning a little."

Nidhi stared at him for a moment and then replied, "At least we're drowning in the same place." Years later, she told me that was the night they truly became partners in parenthood.

The Six-Week Recovery

The Slow Return Toward Yourself. At some point during the sixth week after birth, many women experience a small but important moment. It is rarely dramatic. Perhaps they wake one morning and realise they stood up from bed without pain. Perhaps they walk past a mirror and recognise their own face again beneath the exhaustion. Perhaps they laugh properly for the first time in weeks without feeling physically fragile afterward.

Or perhaps they simply notice that survival no longer requires every ounce of energy. The baby is still waking at night. The house is still disorganised. Laundry still exists in impossible quantities. But something has shifted quietly inside the body. Healing, which once felt invisible, has started becoming noticeable.

This is why the six-week mark matters psychologically as much as medically. It represents the beginning of transition from immediate postpartum survival into gradual adaptation.

Not complete recovery. But the beginning of it.

Why Six Weeks Matters in Medicine

Traditionally, postpartum care has revolved around the "six-week check-up." This timing exists because by six weeks, many major physiological recovery processes have progressed substantially.

By this stage:

- the uterus has usually returned close to pre-pregnancy size,
- lochia has often stopped or become minimal,
- surgical wounds and stitches have significantly healed,
- blood volume has stabilised,
- hormone fluctuations are beginning to settle,
- and the risk of major postpartum complications decreases substantially.

But while medicine often treats six weeks as the endpoint of recovery, many women discover something important at this appointment: They are not fully recovered yet.And that is normal.

YOUR BODY RIGHT NOW

Six weeks postpartum.

Your body has undergone remarkable healing in a short period of time. The uterus has completed most involution. Blood vessels supplying the placenta have sealed and healed. Connective tissue damaged during pregnancy and delivery continues remodeling. Abdominal muscles remain weaker than before pregnancy but are gradually regaining function. Hormonal patterns are stabilising, though breastfeeding may continue suppressing estrogen production for months.

Externally, you may appear "recovered" to other people.

Internally, recovery is still ongoing.

The Postpartum Check-Up

The six-week postpartum visit is one of the most important appointments many women underestimate. During pregnancy, women are monitored constantly: blood pressure, scans, fetal growth, laboratory tests, symptoms, movement counting.

Then suddenly after delivery, medical attention shifts heavily toward the baby. But postpartum health matters enormously too.

This appointment should include:

- physical recovery assessment,
- bleeding review,
- wound healing evaluation,
- contraception discussion,
- pelvic floor symptoms,
- breastfeeding concerns,
- blood pressure assessment,
- emotional wellbeing screening,
- and discussion of any persistent pain or exhaustion.

Many women minimise symptoms at this visit because they assume suffering is "just part of motherhood."

Sometimes it is normal adaptation.

Sometimes it is treatable pathology.

Persistent problems deserve attention.

Pain Is Not Always Normal. By six weeks, severe worsening pain should not be ignored.

Women sometimes silently tolerate:

- persistent pelvic heaviness,
- urinary leakage,
- painful intercourse,
- severe back pain,
- unresolved incision pain,
- bowel problems,
- or emotional numbness

because they believe motherhood requires endurance without complaint.

But postpartum medicine exists because recovery can become complicated. Pelvic floor dysfunction, postpartum thyroiditis, anemia, infection, depression, breastfeeding trauma, and chronic pain syndromes are real medical issues , not personal weakness.

One of the most important shifts modern obstetrics must continue making is this: Women deserve postpartum care, not simply postpartum survival.

My NOTE

I often ask mothers at the six-week visit a question very few people have asked them since delivery:

"How are you ,not the baby ,actually doing?"

Sometimes women answer immediately.

Sometimes they suddenly begin crying.

The postpartum period teaches women to focus so intensely on keeping the baby alive that they often stop monitoring their own wellbeing entirely. But the mother is not secondary to the story.

She is half of it.

The Return of Ordinary Life

Around six weeks, the outside world often begins expecting normal functioning again. Partners return fully to work.

Messages slow down. Visitors stop checking in regularly.

People assume recovery is complete because time has passed.

But internally, many women still feel profoundly changed.

Motherhood alters routine in ways that are difficult to explain to people outside it:

- sleep remains fragmented,
- mental load remains constant,
- feeding continues around the clock,
- and the nervous system remains highly alert to infant needs.

Even leaving the house becomes an organised operation involving diapers, feeding timing, extra clothes, blankets, and contingency planning.

Ordinary life has not fully returned. A different life has begun.

The Body in the Mirror

By six weeks postpartum, some physical changes begin improving noticeably. Swelling decreases. The abdomen becomes firmer. Movement feels easier. Bleeding lessens or stops. The face looks less exhausted. But many women continue struggling emotionally with body image during this stage. Stretch marks remain. Weight may remain. Breasts may feel unfamiliar. Hair may begin shedding. Clothes may fit differently.

And underneath all this is a deeper emotional truth:

The postpartum body carries visible evidence of transformation.

Modern culture often pressures women to erase that evidence quickly to "bounce back," regain shape rapidly, appear unchanged. But biologically, motherhood is not meant to leave the body untouched.

No major physiological event does. The body after childbirth is not ruined. It is experienced.

THE SCIENCE BEHIND IT

Why Recovery Continues Long After Six Weeks

Although six weeks is a traditional medical milestone, connective tissue remodeling, pelvic floor healing, muscular recovery, and hormonal stabilisation continue for many months postpartum.

Breastfeeding may suppress estrogen production for prolonged periods, affecting: mood, vaginal lubrication, bone metabolism, and menstrual cycles.

Sleep deprivation also continues influencing immune and metabolic function long beyond the immediate postpartum phase. In many ways, postpartum recovery is closer to marathon recovery than short-term illness recovery.

The Emotional Shift Around Six Weeks

Something emotional often changes gradually around this stage too.In the beginning, many mothers operate entirely in survival mode: feed the baby, change the baby, sleep briefly, repeat.

But by six weeks, moments of genuine rhythm begin appearing.

The mother starts understanding: different cries, feeding patterns, sleep cues, small personality traits.

The baby no longer feels entirely mysterious. Confidence appears quietly. Not because everything has become easy. But because unfamiliarity is decreasing. This is one of the hidden truths of early motherhood: confidence usually arrives through repetition, not instinct.

The Return of Identity

Around this stage, many women begin asking deeper questions internally.

Who am I now besides someone's mother?

Can I still be:

- ambitious,
- intelligent,
- independent,
- attractive,
- creative,
- social,
- professional,
- myself?

The answer is ***yes***.

But identity after motherhood often becomes layered rather than replaced. Motherhood adds something profound to identity. It does not erase everything that existed before it. Still, adaptation takes time. Some women rediscover themselves quickly. Others take months or years. Neither process is wrong.

The Relationship With the Baby

By six weeks, attachment often deepens in quieter, steadier ways.

In the beginning, love may feel mixed with shock, fear, responsibility, and exhaustion. Now small interactions begin rewarding the parent emotionally: longer eye contact, familiar sounds, calmer feeding, the first social smile approaching in coming weeks.

The baby is slowly becoming a person rather than only a responsibility. And the mother is slowly becoming herself again while also becoming someone new.

The Complicated Beauty of Recovery

There is grief in postpartum recovery sometimes.
Grief for the previous body.
Previous freedom.
Previous simplicity.
Previous identity.

And there is beauty too.
The body heals.
The baby grows.
The family reorganises itself around love and exhaustion and routine and resilience.
One day the mother notices she no longer panics every time the baby cries.
One day she realises she laughed genuinely.
One day she drinks tea while it is still hot.
These things sound small from the outside. Inside early motherhood, they feel enormous.

WHAT YOU MIGHT BE FEELING

At six weeks postpartum, many women exist in a strange middle space no longer in immediate crisis, but not yet fully stable either. There is often relief mixed with lingering exhaustion. Confidence mixed with self-doubt. Increasing emotional attachment mixed with moments of longing for previous independence.

And underneath all of it is gradual adaptation.
Not dramatic, Not perfect, But real.

" Sara's Six-Week Appointment

At her six-week visit, Sara sat quietly while I asked the routine questions about bleeding, feeding, sleep, and healing.
Then I asked, "How are you feeling emotionally?"
She looked surprised for a moment, as though no one had asked her that in weeks.

Finally she said softly, "I think I'm beginning to come back."

I remember smiling at that sentence because it captured postpartum recovery perfectly.

Not suddenly healed. Not exactly the same woman as before.

Just slowly, steadily, returning toward herself while carrying someone new in her arms.

Becoming Yourself Again

The Woman After Motherhood

There is a misconception about motherhood that appears everywhere, in films, family conversations, social media, even sometimes in medicine itself.

The misconception is this: That once a woman becomes a mother, every previous version of herself disappears completely and happily into that role.

Reality is more complicated. Motherhood changes a woman profoundly, but it does not erase her humanity beyond motherhood. Beneath the feeding schedules, school admissions, vaccinations, laundry, and sleepless nights still exists the same person who once had private thoughts, ambitions, fears, humour, desires, friendships, plans, and a life that belonged entirely to herself.

One of the quietest challenges of the postpartum months is learning how to carry both identities simultaneously: the mother, and the woman.

For some women, this balance arrives naturally.

For others, it takes much longer.

Both experiences are normal.

The Disappearance of the Old Life

In the first months after birth, many women experience moments of startling disorientation.

They may look at old photographs and feel as though they belong to someone else. They may hear friends discussing ordinary routines, sleeping late, spontaneous travel, uninterrupted conversations, career plans , and feel unexpectedly emotional.

Not because they regret motherhood. But because major life transitions often involve grief alongside joy.

This is rarely discussed openly because society prefers motherhood to appear emotionally uncomplicated. Women are expected to feel endlessly fulfilled by maternal love alone.

But psychologically, becoming a mother often requires letting go of previous versions of life:

- unrestricted time,
- physical independence,
- spontaneity,
- uninterrupted ambition,
- private space,
- uninterrupted sleep,
- and sometimes parts of identity built over decades.

Even joyful transitions involve loss.

Acknowledging that loss does not make a woman ungrateful.

It makes her honest.

YOUR LIFE RIGHT NOW

Your identity is expanding rather than replacing itself. Neurologically, emotionally, and socially, motherhood is integrating into existing personality structures while also altering priorities, emotional sensitivity, and perception of responsibility. Your brain continues adapting through experience, attachment, repetition, and environmental response.

You are not becoming less yourself.You are becoming a more complicated version of yourself.The Pressure to "Have It All Together"

At some stage after childbirth, women begin encountering subtle pressure to appear fully adjusted.

People ask: "Back to normal now?" "When are you returning to work?" "Have you lost the pregnancy weight?" "Is the baby sleeping through the night yet?" "You must be used to motherhood by now."

These questions often come from harmless curiosity.

But beneath them sits an unrealistic expectation: that adaptation to motherhood should happen quickly and cleanly.

In reality, adjustment is uneven.

A woman may feel emotionally confident with the baby while still struggling physically.

She may return to work professionally while still grieving changes in identity privately.

She may appear composed publicly while crying in the shower from exhaustion at home.

Human adaptation is rarely linear.

My NOTE

One of the most important things I tell new mothers is this:Do not rush to become your "old self" again.That version of you existed before pregnancy, birth, and motherhood. Of course you are changed now. But change is not automatically damage. Sometimes growth feels unfamiliar before it feels strong.

The Relationship With the Body

As months pass, many postpartum physical changes improve gradually. The abdomen strengthens. Hair shedding slows. Sleep sometimes improves. Movement feels easier. Hormones stabilise. But the emotional relationship women have with their bodies after childbirth is often deeper than appearance alone.

The body after pregnancy carries memory. Stretch marks remember stretching. Scars remember surgery. Breasts remember feeding. Pelvic muscles remember pressure and labour.

For some women, these changes become symbols of pride. For others, they remain emotionally complicated for a long time.

Both reactions deserve compassion. What matters most is understanding this: A postpartum body is not evidence of failure to remain unchanged. It is evidence that the body succeeded in doing something extraordinary.

Returning to Work, Study, and Professional Identity

One of the major emotional transitions after early motherhood is returning toward professional or intellectual life.

Many women fear motherhood will permanently reduce their competence, ambition, creativity, or independence.

This fear is understandable because early motherhood temporarily consumes enormous mental bandwidth.

But temporary immersion is not permanent disappearance.

Women often discover something unexpected after motherhood:

- increased emotional resilience,
- sharper prioritisation,
- deeper empathy,
- improved efficiency,
- greater tolerance for stress,
- and a more profound understanding of responsibility.

Motherhood changes professional identity.

It does not automatically diminish it.

Still, returning to work or study after childbirth can feel emotionally complex.

Many women experience:

- guilt leaving the baby,
- guilt enjoying work,
- anxiety about balancing both roles,
- fear of judgment from others regardless of choices made.

There is no universally correct balance.

Every family negotiates this differently.

THE SCIENCE BEHIND IT

The Maternal Brain Continues Changing After Birth.Research using neuroimaging demonstrates that structural and functional changes in the maternal brain continue well beyond pregnancy and delivery.

Areas involved in:

- emotional processing,
- empathy,
- vigilance,
- reward pathways,
- and social bonding shows long-term adaptation during motherhood.

These changes are not signs of cognitive decline.

They represent neurological specialization toward caregiving, emotional attunement, and social responsiveness.

The Friendship Shift

Motherhood often changes friendships too.

Some relationships deepen unexpectedly. Some fade quietly. Some become difficult to maintain simply because time and energy disappear.

Women sometimes feel isolated during this phase because their internal world changes faster than their social environment.

Conversations that once felt important may no longer matter as much. New anxieties emerge. New priorities appear.

And many mothers quietly crave adult conversation unrelated to feeding, sleeping, or diapers.

This longing is healthy.

Motherhood should expand identity, not imprison it.

Learning to Ask for Help

One of the strongest women I know clinically are often the worst at asking for help.

They continue:

- functioning while exhausted,
- smiling while overwhelmed,
- caregiving while depleted.

Modern motherhood frequently rewards self-sacrifice publicly while ignoring its psychological cost privately.But sustainable motherhood requires support.No human nervous system functions well indefinitely under:

- chronic sleep deprivation,
- emotional labour,
- physical caregiving,
- isolation,
- and constant responsibility.

Women deserve:

- rest,
- partnership,
- practical support,
- healthcare,
- nutrition,
- emotional safety,
- and time that belongs occasionally to themselves.

Needing those things does not reduce maternal devotion.

It protects it.

The Unexpected Confidence of Motherhood

Somewhere along the way, often quietly, mothers begin realising something else has changed.

They are stronger than they were before.Not stronger in the dramatic cinematic sense.Stronger in smaller, more enduring ways.

They learn they can function through exhaustion. Protect another human being instinctively. Endure fear and continue anyway. Operate under pressure. Love someone with terrifying intensity. Motherhood humbles women. But it often strengthens them too.

The New Version of Happiness

Before motherhood, happiness may have looked different: achievement,travel,freedom,romance,recognition,ambition fulfilled. After motherhood, happiness often becomes unexpectedly ordinary.

A sleeping baby against your chest. A peaceful feeding. A family meal without chaos. A shower uninterrupted. Your child is smiling when they see you enter the room.

These moments would once have seemed insignificant.

Now they feel immense. Not because motherhood lowers standards for joy. Because it changes attention.

WHAT YOU MIGHT BE FEELING

As the postpartum months continue, many women begin feeling emotionally steadier while also confronting deeper questions about identity, ambition, relationships, body image, and purpose. There is often relief that survival has become easier, mixed with uncertainty about how to integrate motherhood into the rest of life rather than allowing it to consume everything.

And slowly, almost invisibly, confidence begins replacing fear.

Not because motherhood becomes simple.

But because unfamiliarity decreases.

You stop feeling like someone pretending to be a mother.

You begin realising you are one.

" Isha's Realisation

One afternoon, several months after delivery, Isha sat drinking tea while her son slept beside her.

For the first time since childbirth, the house was quiet.

She looked down at the stretch marks across her abdomen and said softly, almost to herself, "I spent months trying to get my old life back."

Then she smiled faintly.

"But I don't think I'm meant to go backward anymore."

Years later she told me that was the moment motherhood stopped feeling like an interruption to her identity and started feeling like part of it.

Healthy Pregnancy Essentials

Simple Things That Protect Both Mother and Baby

Pregnancy does not require perfection.It requires consistency.

Across years of obstetric practice, I have noticed something reassuring: healthy pregnancies are usually built not from dramatic interventions, but from small daily habits repeated patiently over many months. Eating regularly. Taking supplements. Attending check-ups. Resting when tired. Listening to the body instead of fighting against it.

Women are often overwhelmed during pregnancy by endless advice from relatives, social media, neighbours, and the internet. Some advice is helpful. Much of it is confusing. This chapter is not about complicated rules. It is about the essentials that genuinely matter medically for a safer and healthier pregnancy.

The most important thing to understand is this:

Your body already knows how to grow a baby.
Your job is not to control every detail perfectly.
Your job is to support the process wisely.

What To Do During Pregnancy

Attend your antenatal visits regularly, even when you feel completely fine. Many pregnancy complications such as high blood pressure, gestational diabetes, anaemia, fetal growth restriction, and thyroid disorders may develop silently before symptoms appear. Regular check-ups allow problems to be identified early, when treatment is most effective.

Take folic acid, iron, calcium, and prescribed supplements consistently. Supplements only work when taken regularly. Iron helps prevent anaemia and supports fetal oxygen delivery. Calcium supports fetal skeletal development while protecting maternal bone stores. Folic acid significantly reduces neural tube defects. Vitamin D, increasingly important in Indian women due to widespread deficiency, supports bone health and immune function.

Sleep whenever your body asks for rest. Pregnancy fatigue is physiological, not laziness. Blood volume expands dramatically during pregnancy, metabolism increases, hormonal changes intensify, and the cardiovascular system works continuously to support placental circulation. Rest is part of treatment.

Stay physically active with safe moderate exercise. Walking, prenatal yoga, stretching, and gentle mobility exercises improve circulation, reduce constipation, decrease excessive weight gain, improve mood, lower gestational diabetes risk, and often make labour easier. The body is designed for movement during uncomplicated pregnancy.

Drink enough water. Pregnancy increases blood volume, amniotic fluid production, kidney workload, and metabolic demand. Dehydration can worsen headaches, constipation, dizziness, urinary infections, and uterine irritability.

Learn your baby's movement pattern in the second half of pregnancy. Babies have sleep cycles and active periods, but a noticeable reduction in movements always deserves medical attention. Maternal awareness of fetal movement remains one of the simplest and most powerful ways to recognise fetal distress early.

Take care of your emotional health with the same seriousness as physical health. Anxiety, loneliness, depression, fear, and emotional exhaustion are common during pregnancy and deserve support, not silence.

What To Avoid During Pregnancy

Avoid ***smoking*** completely. Cigarette smoke reduces oxygen delivery to the baby and significantly increases risks of miscarriage, placental complications, low birth weight, preterm birth, stillbirth, and sudden infant death syndrome.

Avoid ***alcohol*** entirely during pregnancy. No safe amount has been clearly established. Alcohol crosses the placenta directly and may affect fetal brain development at every stage of pregnancy.

Avoid ***self-medication***. Many common medicines – including painkillers, antibiotics, hormonal drugs, and herbal preparations may affect pregnancy. Always discuss medications with your doctor before taking them.

Avoid excessive ***caffeine***. Moderate tea or coffee intake is usually acceptable, but very high caffeine intake has been associated with increased miscarriage risk and fetal growth concerns. Balance matters.

Avoid ***unpasteurised dairy products***, undercooked meat, raw eggs, and unhygienically prepared street foods during pregnancy because foodborne infections can become dangerous for both mother and fetus.

Avoid ***extreme dieting or "eating for two."*** Pregnancy requires nutritional quality more than excessive quantity. Rapid unhealthy weight gain increases risks of gestational diabetes, hypertension, difficult labour, and cesarean delivery.

Avoid ***comparing your pregnancy*** constantly with others. Every pregnancy behaves differently. Some women vomit daily. Some never experience nausea. Some develop visible bumps early. Others carry small throughout pregnancy. Variation is normal.

What To Eat During Pregnancy

A healthy pregnancy diet does not require expensive imported foods or complicated meal plans.

Traditional balanced Indian meals, when prepared thoughtfully, are often nutritionally excellent.

Focus on:
- protein, iron, calcium,fibre,hydration, and balanced energy intake.

Protein is essential because fetal tissues, placenta, maternal blood volume, and breast tissue all require continuous protein synthesis during pregnancy. Good sources include dal, paneer, curd, milk, eggs, fish, chicken, sprouts, soy products, nuts, and legumes.

Iron-rich foods include green leafy vegetables, jaggery, dates, beetroot, lentils, black chana, rajma, pomegranate, meat, and liver where culturally appropriate. Combining iron-rich foods with Vitamin C sources such as lemon or amla improves absorption significantly.

Calcium-rich foods include milk, curd, paneer, ragi, sesame seeds, almonds, and leafy greens. Calcium becomes increasingly important during the second and third trimesters when fetal bone mineralisation accelerates.

Fresh fruits and vegetables provide fibre, antioxidants, hydration, and micronutrients essential for maternal bowel health, immunity, and fetal development.

Healthy fats from nuts, seeds, ghee in moderation, and traditional home-cooked meals support fetal brain development and maternal hormonal health.

Frequent small meals often work better than large heavy meals, especially during nausea and late pregnancy reflux.

What To Watch For During Pregnancy

Certain symptoms during pregnancy always deserve medical attention and should never be ignored.

Seek medical care immediately if you experience:

heavy bleeding, leaking fluid, severe abdominal pain, persistent vomiting with dehydration, severe headache, blurred vision, swelling of face and hands, reduced fetal movements, breathlessness, fever, chest pain, seizures, or high blood pressure readings.

Many serious pregnancy complications become manageable when recognised early.

Delaying medical care out of fear, social pressure, or assumptions that symptoms are "normal" can become dangerous.

Trust your instincts.

Mothers often recognise that something feels wrong before laboratory tests confirm it.

A Final Thought

Pregnancy is not only the growth of a baby. It is the gradual formation of a mother. Some days you will feel strong, Some days frightened. Some days deeply connected to the experience. Some days simply tired.

All of those days belong to real pregnancy.

You do not need to become a perfect pregnant woman.

You only need to care for yourself with patience, consistency, and kindness while your body performs one of the most extraordinary biological processes in human life.

Golden ANTENATAL ADVICE

- Attend ALL scheduled antenatal visits, do not skip even if feeling well
- Take prescribed medications regularly; never self-medicate during pregnancy
- Absolutely avoid alcohol, smoking, tobacco, gutkha, and recreational drugs throughout pregnancy
- Maintain good perineal hygiene; wear clean cotton underwear; report unusual vaginal discharge
- Sleep on your LEFT SIDE from 28 weeks, improves placental blood flow
- Maintain healthy weight gain: total 11–16 kg (normal BMI); 7–11 kg (overweight); 5–9 kg (obese)
- Wear seat belt during travel: lap belt below bump; shoulder belt between breasts
- Do NOT travel to high-altitude destinations or fly after 36 weeks without obstetric clearance
- Mental health: report persistent sadness, anxiety, panic attacks to your doctor ,Perinatal Mental Health matters
- Breastfeed exclusively for 6 months after birth, protects baby against infections, SIDS, and promotes bonding
- Register under Janani Suraksha Yojana (JSY) / PMSMA for institutional delivery benefits
- Emergency Helpline: 108 (Ambulance) | Janani Express available 24x7 in Madhya Pradesh

Message from the Author

There is a saying, "You will truly understand it only when it happens to you." During my own pregnancy, I realized how true these words are.

As an obstetrician and gynecologist, I had cared for thousands of pregnant women. I understood pregnancy from a medical point of view. But when I became pregnant myself, I experienced the physical changes, emotional ups and downs, hopes, fears, and joys that every expectant mother goes through. This journey gave me a new perspective and an even deeper respect for every mother.

This book is my humble effort to combine scientific knowledge with my personal experiences. I have written it in simple language so that everyone can understand pregnancy better. It includes evidence-based information for general awareness, along with the lessons I learned during my own journey, from the day I discovered I was pregnant until I returned to my clinical duties.

I hope this book helps expectant mothers feel informed, confident, and supported. I also hope it helps fathers, grandparents, family members, medical students, and healthcare professionals better understand the beautiful journey of pregnancy.

Thank you for choosing this book. It is not only for mothers, it is for everyone who wishes to understand, support, and celebrate the journey of bringing a new life into the world.

With gratitude,

Dr. Babita Das
MBBS, MS (Obstetrics & Gynecology)

"Compassion and Science together create safer Pregnancies."

Notes

REFERENCES AND FURTHER READING

1. Williams Obstetrics. 26th ed. New York: McGraw-Hill Education; 2022.

2. Konar H. DC Dutta's Textbook of Obstetrics. 10th ed. New Delhi: Jaypee Brothers Medical Publishers; 2023.

3. Daftary SN, Chakravarti S. Shaw's Textbook of Gynecology. 18th ed. New Delhi: Elsevier India; 2023.

4. Berek JS. Berek & Novak's Gynecology. 16th ed. Philadelphia: Wolters Kluwer; 2020.

5. Gabbe SG, Niebyl JR, Simpson JL, et al. Obstetrics: Normal and Problem Pregnancies. 8th ed. Philadelphia: Elsevier; 2021.

6. Resnik R, Lockwood CJ, Moore TR, Greene MF, Copel JA, Silver RM. Creasy and Resnik's Maternal-Fetal Medicine: Principles and Practice. 9th ed. Philadelphia: Elsevier; 2023.

7. Hacker NF, Gambone JC, Hobel CJ. Hacker & Moore's Essentials of Obstetrics and Gynecology. 7th ed. Philadelphia: Elsevier; 2022.

8. DeCherney AH, Nathan L, Laufer N, Roman AS. Current Diagnosis & Treatment: Obstetrics & Gynecology. 12th ed. New York: McGraw-Hill Education.

9. Edmonds DK. Dewhurst's Textbook of Obstetrics and Gynaecology. 9th ed. Wiley-Blackwell.

10. Marshall JE, Raynor MD. Myles Textbook for Midwives. 17th ed. Elsevier; 2020.

11. World Health Organization (WHO). WHO Recommendations on Antenatal Care for a Positive Pregnancy Experience.

13. World Health Organization (WHO). Recommendations on Maternal and Newborn Care for a Positive Postnatal Experience.

14. American College of Obstetricians and Gynecologists (ACOG). Practice Bulletins and Committee Opinions.

15. Royal College of Obstetricians and Gynaecologists (RCOG). Green-top Guidelines.

16. International Society of Ultrasound in Obstetrics and Gynecology (ISUOG). Practice Guidelines.

17. Federation of Obstetric and Gynaecological Societies of India (FOGSI). Good Clinical Practice Recommendations.

18. Indian Council of Medical Research (ICMR). Maternal Health and Nutrition Guidelines.

19. Ministry of Health and Family Welfare, Government of India. RMNCH+A Strategy and Maternal Health Guidelines.

20. National Institute for Health and Care Excellence (NICE). Antenatal, Intrapartum and Postnatal Care Guidelines.

"Protecting Mothers, Empowering Women."

www.ingramcontent.com/pod-product-compliance
Lightning Source LLC
LaVergne TN
LVHW100253210926
848480LV00003B/916